Qualitative Research in Health and Illness

Qualitative Research in Health and Illness

Jessica Smartt Gullion

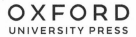

OXFORD
UNIVERSITY PRESS

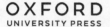

Oxford University Press is a department of the University of Oxford. It furthers the University's objective of excellence in research, scholarship, and education by publishing worldwide. Oxford is a registered trade mark of Oxford University Press in the UK and certain other countries.

Published in the United States of America by Oxford University Press
198 Madison Avenue, New York, NY 10016, United States of America.

Library of Congress Cataloging-in-Publication Data
Names: Gullion, Jessica Smartt, author.
Title: Qualitative research in health and illness / Jessica Smartt Gullion, PhD.
Description: New York, NY : Oxford University Press, [2024] |
Series: Research to the point | Includes bibliographical references and index. |
Identifiers: LCCN 2023038926 (print) | LCCN 2023038927 (ebook) |
ISBN 9780197769638 (pb) | ISBN 9780190915988 (hb) | ISBN 9780190916008 (epub) |
ISBN 9780190916015 (ebook)
Subjects: LCSH: Public health—Research—Methodology. |
Health—Research—Methodology. | Medicine—Research—Methodology. |
Qualitative research.
Classification: LCC RA440.85 .S593 2024 (print) | LCC RA440.85 (ebook) |
DDC 362.1072—dc23/eng/20230925
LC record available at https://lccn.loc.gov/2023038926
LC ebook record available at https://lccn.loc.gov/2023038927

DOI: 10.1093/oso/9780190915988.001.0001

Paperback printed by Marquis Book Printing, Canada
Hardback printed by Bridgeport National Bindery, Inc., United States of America

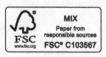

Contents

Acknowledgments

I am grateful that my academic career unfolded nonlinearly. After graduation with my PhD in sociology, I had the opportunity to serve as the Chief Epidemiologist at the Denton County Health Department (which covers a population of about three quarters of a million people). I owe a debt of gratitude to those public health workers who trained me and showed me just how qualitative epidemiology and health research need to be. When it comes to their health, people don't think linearly, and unforeseen variables (such as a case of cheap beer, a gun, and a skunk) enter into the equations that predict health outcomes.

Qualitative Research in Health and Illness was written at the generous invitation of Dr Patricia Leavy and Oxford University Press. This is the fourth book I've had the honor of writing for one of Dr Leavy's book series. I am so grateful for our friendship; Patricia is a feminist powerhouse and I am privileged to call her my friend. Feminist fist bump to you and to Sandra Faulkner for your encouragement and sanity before and during the coronapocalypse. Thank you also to Abby Gross for your support of this project.

I would also like to acknowledge my writing group and the baristas at Cryptozoology for the flow of support and caffeine. I'm so sorry Crypto did not weather the COVID-19 storm. Thanks also to Abigail Tilton, Claire Sahlin, Shannon Scott, Holly Hansen-Thomas for your on-going support of my work. Thank you to Donna Scott-Tilley for inviting me to your writing retreat—getting away was re-energizing.

And as always, thank you to Greg, Renn, and Rory for all of your love, support, and a steady supply of nachos.

I wrote this book during the COVID-19 pandemic. These were some of the most turbulent years of my life. In addition to personal events and difficulties, COVID-19 raged across the U.S. (at the time of this writing having cause more than one million deaths) and changed everything—how we do work, school, how we live life. COVID killed several of my friends, and I attended my first (surreal, postapocalyptic) Zoom funeral. I thank everyone who supported me in all their different ways through this time of collective trauma. My anthem has been The Mountain Goats' song, *This Year*: "I am going to make it through this year if it kills me." COVID-19 left us with plenty of research to do.

About the Author

Jessica Smartt Gullion, PhD, is Associate Dean of Research for the College of Arts and Sciences and Professor of Sociology at Texas Woman's University. She has written extensively on social science methodology and in the field of medical sociology.

Other Books by the Author

Nonfiction

Diffractive Ethnography: Social Sciences and the Ontological Turn
Fracking the Neighborhood: Reluctant Activists and Natural Gas Drilling
Writing Ethnography (now in its second edition)
Researching With: A Decolonizing Approach to Community-Based Action Research (with Abigail Tilton)

Anthologies

Redefining Disability (with Paul Bones and Danielle Barber)
In Sickness and Health: Sociological Perspectives on Healthcare (with John Malek-Ahmadi)
Voices in Sociology: An Introduction to the Core Concepts (with Cynthia T. Cook, Helen Brethauer-Gay, and Amitra Hodge-Wall)

Fiction

October Birds

Abbreviations

AAUP	American Association of University Professors
ADA	Americans with Disabilities Act
ASL	American Sign Language
CFP	calls for proposals
COVID-19	Coronavirus Disease 2019
CRT	critical race theory
FERPA	Family Educational Rights and Privacy Act
HIPAA	Health Insurance Portability and Accountability Act
HIV	human immunodeficiency virus
IDC	indirect costs
IRB	institutional review board
NIH	National Institutes of Health
ORSP	Office of Research and Sponsored Programs
PI	principal investigator
PPRA	Protection of Pupil Rights Amendment (No Child Left Behind)
PRISMA	Preferred Reporting Items for Systematic Reviews and Meta-Analysis
PTSA	parent–teacher–student association
SANE	Sexual Assault Nurse Examiners

Introduction

"Hands on hips, smiles on lips ladies," the coach shouted as the girls marched up to the stage. I scribbled the sentence into the small notebook that I had brought with me to this cheerleading competition. Sometimes it's hard to know what to write down when you're doing ethnographic fieldwork; other times something like this stands out as an important detail.

I am a qualitative researcher. I find people's actions fascinating and wonderfully complex. And scenes like this, scenes that feel so pertinent to an overall project, can only be captured in the social sciences by using qualitative data collection.

I have conducted and taught qualitative research methods for most of my professional life. The data that a researcher can collect using qualitative techniques are rich and complex, and they can give deep insights into the social world. I wrote this book to provide you with an accessible, pragmatic approach to conducting qualitative research in the health fields, whether you are conducting research in a health care setting, in public health, or in the community. Targeted toward novice researchers, I provide tools to address scenarios that are likely to arise during the course of your research. To do this, I will lead you through some of the common methods of data collection and analysis that qualitative researchers use.

I take a broad view of practices that could fall under the heading of qualitative inquiry. Any empirical materials (i.e., data) that do not begin as numeric could fall into this heading. I prefer to keep qualitative inquiry as a concept open-ended in order to widen the possibilities for what we can do as researchers rather than confine the parameters. By this I mean that there are many ways of doing qualitative research and that we should not restrict ourselves to one or two methods that we believe are the "right way" to understand the world. This opening means you may be presented with contradictions and tensions as you learn about different approaches to research. That's ok; this gives you different tools for different situations. This being said, we will review a number of established qualitative methods that can be put to immediate use.

Qualitative Research in Health and Illness. Jessica Smartt Gullion, Oxford University Press. © Oxford University Press 2024.
DOI: 10.1093/oso/9780190915988.003.0001

Although there are perspectives that resonate more with me than others, in this book I give you a broad toolbox to work with. This may at times feel disjointed, as some authors write in opposition to each other. It is important for you to sit with the material, engage supplementary texts, and determine what method works best both for you and for your project.

I present a variety of data collection and analytic techniques, but it is important to note that many volumes could be (and, indeed, are) dedicated to each of these individually and that there are other techniques that I do not cover. While I intend for this book to be used to guide your work, I also encourage you to read broadly about the methods you choose to use. You will not get an adequate understanding of any method from one textbook; you need to read many examples of that type of work and find what works best for your particular situation.

In addition, an important caveat that should be placed in all methods textbooks is that none of what the author writes is prescriptive. All of the techniques and methods we introduce were created at different times to serve different purposes. These techniques have since been tested, debated, and refined; however, you may find a need to adapt, refurbish, or even invent new methods for your own particular situation. As we will see later in this book, this is why you need to explain in the written account of your research exactly what you did and why, so your reader can understand your process and judge your work accordingly.

Research in real life is never as straightforward as it seems in textbooks. The structure of writing about method makes it seem like method is a stepwise, linear process. I want to emphasize that this is not the case at all. Research is more often messy and chaotic, and you will often find yourself going back and forth among and between steps. Research is *hard*. But the journey is also incredibly rewarding.

There are times when you need research methods to answer a particular, matter-of-fact question. For example, you might want to know what barriers patients have to taking their medications as prescribed, or what happens during patient care to increase hospital-associated infections. Other times, you may be interested in deeper philosophical questions, such as the ontology of a disease, or refining a theory of health behavior. In both cases, you can use techniques in this book to build your understanding and answer the questions you have about health and illness.

While you will find many suggestions of how to do research, examples of how others have done research, and ways that scholars have refined research techniques, research methods should be fluid. Many students would prefer a "how to" manual, but in real life, no matter what others tell you, research seldom follows prescriptive rules. I invite you to leave the door open, hone your creative and intellectual skills, and find what works best for you and for your research.

If you have decided to be a qualitative researcher because "statistics are hard," I've got some bad news for you. Although there are some wonderful software packages out there to help you manage data, they won't do the analysis for you. Qualitative research requires deep thought, and thinking is hard. Research is complicated. There is no computer program that will spit out the "right" answer for you. Nothing to tell you the answer is 42 and significant at the $p < .05$ level. When qualitative research is done well, it is difficult and demanding. It is also a gratifying way to spend your career.

Overview of the Text

There are three parts to this text. In Part I, we explore the foundations of qualitative research. This includes a basic overview of what qualitative research is and what it can help you to do. We spend a large amount of time reviewing the ethics of human subjects research and ways to ensure that our work is done ethically. This includes extra attention for special populations (e.g., pregnant people, children, and prisoners) and how to navigate legal protections about privacy (including HIPPA in the United States). Next, we turn to research design, which includes how to review the literature on your research topic, how to choose a method that is appropriate for your project, and how to make decisions on who and what to include in your research. This section of the book concludes with a discussion about objectivity and researcher standpoint, and the importance of interrogating how you as the researcher might influence that outcome of your research.

Part II of the book focuses on the collection of empirical materials or data. We begin with the most common qualitative data technique: interviewing. I provide a lot of advice on how to interview, and how to interview well. Next, we look at ethnographic techniques of observation and participation and fieldwork. This includes fieldwork on the internet. After that, we take a deep dive into community-based action research, which is where a lot of health education programming and social change activities happen. Then we spend some time exploring medical narratives and storytelling.

In Part III, we discuss different ways to analyze data and write our findings. This includes a discussion of data management, coding, grounded theory, situational analysis, diffraction, and poetic analysis. We conclude the section on analysis with an overview of post-qualitative inquiry. Then we focus on writing up the results of all our hard work, whether we are writing a traditional, scientific report or trying to write for different types of audiences.

Many qualitative researchers, including myself, work in the liminal space where science and art overlap. There's a false dichotomy between the social sciences and the humanities (Faulkner 2020), which is unfortunate because we miss out on interesting ways of working with people and interacting with our data and findings. In this book, we explore how we can use both science and art to expand our understanding and open ways of thinking about research that we may not have previously considered.

A Note for Instructors

This book is intended to be used as a core text in courses in general research methods or qualitative methods courses in the health fields. This includes courses in nursing, health studies, kinesiology, public health, physical/occupational therapy, health care administration, nutrition, medical sociology, and medical anthropology, among others. As I aimed for accessibility over obfuscation, it can be used at both the upper level undergraduate and graduate levels. This book can also be used by health care practitioners and faculty interested in learning how to conduct qualitative research.

I have taught a variety of research methods courses myself, for more than a decade, at both the undergraduate and graduate levels. I am familiar with the types of students who would be using this book, their backgrounds, and the knowledge they already hold when they are introduced to this material.

To aid with instruction, at the end of each chapter I include a brief recommended additional readings list for students who wish to delve deeper into the nuances of the topics they learned, discussion questions for the classroom, active learning assignments, and mindfulness exercises that students can use to journal and reflect on what they are learning. I have also included pop-out boxes with definitions of key terms as students encounter them, and a glossary at the back of the book to assist students who may be encountering new terminology.

Reference

Faulkner, Sandra L. 2020. *Poetic Inquiry: Craft, Method and Practice*, 2nd ed. London: Routledge.

PART I

The Foundations of Qualitative Inquiry

What Is Qualitative Research?

In this chapter, we explore what qualitative research entails and why researchers might want to employ its methods. We begin with a brief history of the emergence of qualitative inquiry. Next, we address some of the common misconceptions about qualitative research. We transition to an overview of ontology (what is reality) and epistemology (how we know a thing) and discuss why understanding our own ontological and epistemological preferences is important when approaching how we conduct research. We review the use of theory, which is followed by a discussion of decolonizing research.

Prior to becoming a professor, I worked as the Chief Epidemiologist at one of the largest health departments in Texas. During my tenure there, I discovered that although I enjoyed quantitative research (my primary focus in graduate school had been nonlinear dynamics in time-series data, which involved a whole lot of number-crunching), qualitative research helped me better understand how communicable diseases spread and develop effective interventions for disease prevention.

Qualitative researchers use text, images, and other non-numeric materials as data.

One morning I received a phone call from a school nurse, reporting that one of the students at her high school was hospitalized with meningococcal meningitis. This is the form of bacterial meningitis that students are vaccinated for. As a preventive measure, all of the student's family members had received an injection of antibiotics. Because household members are considered close exposures, this would kill any of the bacteria they might be incubating and keep them from coming down with the disease. My job as a public health epidemiologist was to identify anyone else who was exposed to the student and make sure they received prophylactic treatment (the antibiotic) as well.

Qualitative Research in Health and Illness. Jessica Smartt Gullion, Oxford University Press. © Oxford University Press 2024.
DOI: 10.1093/oso/9780190915988.003.0002

Meningococcal meningitis is spread via saliva. Normally, I would interview the patient to find out who they may have spent lots of time with, kissed, shared a drink with, and so on. But this patient was on a ventilator. I couldn't interview her.

Of all of the infectious diseases that I worked on, meningococcal meningitis raised the most alarm. A patient could go from lively and vibrant to dead in twenty-four hours. Patients who received treatment early still suffered terrible sequelae (long-term consequences of the disease). Meningococcal meningitis can cause necrosis of the extremities. One patient whom I worked with had all her limbs amputated as a result of her infection. Another lost all of her fingers on one hand and the tip of her nose. While I couldn't do anything to help the girl in the hospital, I could prevent others from going through the same experience. If I could get antibiotics to people who had been exposed to her while she was infectious, I could potentially save their lives.

I drove to the high school to do some investigating. I took a standardized survey instrument with me to administer to the students.

The survey consisted of a number of yes/no questions, such as, Did you kiss the patient? or, Did you smoke a cigarette or any type of pipe with the patient?—a whole list of questions that could determine if someone had a high likelihood of contracting the disease. If a person answered yes to any of the questions, they needed to receive prophylaxis as soon as possible.

I met with the school nurse and principal. They decided the safest thing to do was to shelter the students in place and administer the survey to the entire school. Not all administrators would have taken such bold action, but neither of them could bear the thought of another child getting sick and possibly dying. Although student health information is normally protected and kept private, public health laws allow some information to be shared in order to prevent the spread of disease. The school administrators decided the best course of action was to share the ill student's name.

The principal made an announcement about the incident over the school's intercom. Students were told to remain in their classrooms. The teachers administered the survey orally, and students responded to the questions on paper. Students who marked yes to any one of the survey items were sent by their teachers to the principal's office, where the school nurse and I explained the situation and called their parents to make sure they received treatment.

Eleven students came to the office. I asked them to tell me more about the patient to make sure we'd found everyone who needed treatment. I asked about the patient's after-school and extracurricular activities and found out that the patient played trombone in the school marching band.

I remembered from my own high school band days that the horn players often cleaned their spit valves in class (even though they weren't supposed to; I remembered puddles of spit on the band hall floor). I went to see the band director. He agreed that sometimes the students still did this. Luckily for us, band members are assigned chairs in the band hall based on their skill level, and they always sit in the same spot. The band director and I identified six students who sat in close enough vicinity to the patient that I recommended they receive treatment. None of these six answered yes to any of the questions on the survey.

The band director mentioned that the brass players received new mouthpieces for their horns that week. They tried out each other's mouthpieces, and the ill girl took part in this. We found several more exposed teens.

These teenagers had been exposed to a life-threatening illness, preventable with medication, but they were not identified with the survey. Instead, they were helped with the use of qualitative methods—by talking to people, and learning about their lives in ways that surveys don't capture.

This experience solidified the importance of qualitative research for me. My quantitative survey identified some of the people in need of treatment; qualitative inquiry identified more. When it comes to people's health, we have to consider the complexity of human behavior and talk with people to understand details that are missed with surveys.

Research methods are the techniques used to conduct research. Social scientists have developed all sorts of tools—surveys, experiments, interviews, focus groups, content analysis, ethnography, and so on—to help us understand human behavior. Each tool informs us about some aspect of the phenomena that we are studying. No one tool tells us everything we might want to know; in fact, many researchers use multiple tools in their research to triangulate their data (this is usually called mixed methods).

> Research methods are the techniques that researchers use to study the social world.

In this text, we explore tools that are qualitative in nature. Qualitative researchers capture and retell stories (Denzin 2010). Often these stories are used to solve problems, such as in the epidemiologic investigation I wrote about earlier. In this book, we examine how to use qualitative methods with research questions derived from health and illness, but qualitative methods can be used to study any aspect of human behavior.

Qualitative research methods treat non-numeric empirical materials as data. Stated differently, qualitative researchers use words, images, sounds, video, and other data that have not been reduced to numbers to understand some research question of interest. This could include activities such as interviewing people, analyzing photographs, exploring the content of websites, reviewing patient charts, viewing educational videos and other materials—so many items can be data for qualitative research.

Humans are constantly bombarded with information, and we make sense of much of that information without thinking too much about it. Information that comes to us in the form of numbers is called quantitative. Information that comes to us in any other form is qualitative. In this book, we explore how to collect information for use in research and how to systematically interact with that data to conduct analysis and write what we've learned to share with others.

We receive input from and about the world continually, and that information comes to us in a variety of forms. When I turn on my morning shower, the water starts off cold. I know it is hot when I touch the stream with my hand and feel that the temperature is where I want it to be. This is a qualitative way of knowing that the shower is ready. I could, if I wanted to, attach a thermometer to my showerhead that read the exact temperature of the water. I could watch the thermometer, and when it reached the temperature I wanted, I could get in the shower. That's a quantitative way of knowing the shower is ready.

One way of knowing the shower is the right temperature for me is not better or worse than the other. They are both valid ways of knowing that I can get in without freezing.

Some academics will try to argue that a qualitative approach is better than a quantitative one, or the reverse, that quantitative methods are superior. Both groups of academics are wrong. While one method might be better to answer a particular research question, qualitative and quantitative methods are simply different ways of knowing; one is not superior to the other. You may find methods that you prefer; we all tend to do that. But you should have a wide range of tools to choose from because different questions invite different methods in order to answer them. You should also be able to read and understand research that others have produced, regardless of the methods they used.

Often, researchers find themselves in allegiance to one camp of research methods that they prefer to work with. Typically, this is qualitative or quantitative, but it could also be more specific—maybe they see themselves aligned with experiments, or ethnography, or they prefer arts-based research methods. While it is good to have in-depth knowledge of one method, you must be careful that such allegiances don't dictate how you go about conducting inquiry, as opposed to allowing the research question to guide how you go about the inquiry. We want methods to open up possibilities, not close them. Gane (2011: 152) argues that this tendency to align with one way of knowing has led to a "crisis of methodological invention." Empiricism becomes abstracted, method becomes standardized, and the whole system becomes rigid and inflexible (Gane 2011; Gullion 2018).

It makes sense that we would be more likely to turn to a method that is more comfortable to us to answer our questions about whatever it is we want to know more about. But that does not necessarily lead to the best research.

> We need to interrogate how to best answer our research questions. Sometimes this might involve having to learn (or even invent) new techniques.

History of Social Science Methods

At some universities, qualitative methods are treated as niche, new, or alternative. Yet the foundational works in the study of human behavior were qualitative studies; quantitative research methods developed more recently.

In this section, I refer specifically to anthropology and sociology because the techniques I refer to in this text were developed and refined in these academic disciplines. Newer disciplines within the social sciences either broke off from one of these two disciplines as a distinct area or they have adopted methods developed by anthropologists or sociologists. This overview is brief; students wanting more in-depth discussion of this history can find some resources at the end of this chapter.

Before the development of quantitative methods, social scientists immersed themselves in the settings they wished to know more about in order to gather data in a systematic way. This type of research is known as ethnography, and it is a useful way of gathering in-depth understanding of phenomena of interest.

The earliest ethnographic accounts were travelogs. Although we would not consider them to be systematic research today, travelogs were used to help people understand a little about other cultures before systematic research methods were developed. Travelogs consisted of notes and stories about the places the author visited.

Anthropologists began to systematize ethnographic methods, transitioning the travelog into science. The British Society for the Advancement of Science published *Notes and Queries on Anthropology, or A Guide to Anthropological Research for the Use of Travelers and Others*[1] in 1874. This is an interesting example of the types of data fieldworkers collected (Erickson 2018: 38–39). It was a little workbook that provided instructions for how to conduct anthropological research, including directions and worksheets for collecting anatomical observations; physical and psychological observations; clothing and ornamentation; housing; transportation; techniques for making clothing, pottery, art, and other goods; food, agriculture, hunting, and food preparation; religious and spiritual beliefs and rituals; morality and customs; laws, crime, and punishment; music and ceremony; language; and a host of other data. It is important to note here that this research was done on a group of people other than the social group the researcher belonged to.

By the early 1900s, anthropologists were engaged in systematic inquiry into what they considered to be "exotic" or "primitive" peoples. To prove themselves, these anthropologists traveled to remote settings. Their overarching goal was to understand how humans in the West evolved from primitive cultures to civilizations. They generally lived among the people under study for long periods of time and used field notes to make sense of the cultural norms they witnessed. They believed it was the job of the researcher to observe, record, categorize, and theorize, primarily about Indigenous peoples (Gullion 2018). The idea was that they could model how societies "evolved" from "primitive" to "civilized." Erickson (2018: 39) cites W. E. B. DuBois' 1899 monograph, *The Philadelphia Negro*, as the first modern realist ethnography. The text did more than catalog; it also advocated for social reform. Many other scholars, however, cite Malinowski's 1922 book, *Argonauts of the Western Pacific*, as the foundational ethnographic text because of its interpretive quality and its descriptions of local meaning—that is, the meanings that the people he studied placed on things and phenomena (MacDonald 2001).

Around this same time, a group of anthropologists that included Franz Boas and his students, Margaret Mead, Ruth Benedict, Ella Cara Deloria, and Zora Neal Hurston, began what they called cultural anthropology, which posited that there was no real difference between groups of humans (King 2019: 5). The general conception at the time was that there was a "natural ranking" of humans and that some groups of humans had simply not yet evolved. Boas and his students set out to show that "the social categories into which we typically divide ourselves, including labels such as race and gender, are at base artificial" (King 2019: 7). This was a radical notion at the time. Rather than viewing different cultures as somehow less than their own, these researchers were more interested in the ways in which cultures differed.

In contrast to the anthropologists, early sociologists tended to study "deviant" populations in the cities in which they lived, or tried to capture "everyday life," which they called social ecology (usually that ecology was composed of groups of people with less social capital—money, status, and education—than the researcher). This was largely due to the influence of the Chicago School, a group of sociologists from the University of Chicago who conducted research in the city. These sociologists were often grounded in the theories of symbolic interactionism; that is, they were interested in how people made meaning. From 1892 through 1942, the Chicago School dominated U.S. sociology. This included scholars such as Park, Burgess, Thomas, Mead, Dewey, and their students (Deegan 2001; Gullion 2018). Their writing tended to be journalistic in style, and projects included topics such as collective behavior, juvenile delinquency, gangs, crime, race relations, the lives of immigrants, and the homeless.

As mentioned previously, these scholars turned to symbolic interactionism, particularly the work of Mead, to situate their work. One of Mead's primary concerns was how people understand, differentiate, and embrace their social roles (Deegan 2001: 19). In later years, this approach would evolve into identity theories—theories about constructs such as race, gender, and sexuality, along with other categories. Their data included detailed field notes, mapping, direct observations, use of participants' diaries, and interviewing. Because the researcher lived and/or worked alongside the people they studied, they tended to use participant observation as their main research method. They became "part of the group" and engaged in the activities of the group in order to better understand them. They were prolific book publishers (the Chicago School benefitted largely from the University of Chicago Press).

In the case of both early anthropology and sociology, there were distinct asymmetries between the researcher and the people being observed (Atkinson et al. 2001).

For the most part, anthropologists today have stuck with ethnographic methods to do their research (although there are quantitative anthropologists). They grapple with how to ensure their work is ethical and decolonizing. Sociologists, in contrast, veered over to quantitative methods with the development of population-based surveys and statistical analysis. This gained traction after World War II (Maynes, Piece, and Laslett 2008). Using quantitative methods, sociologists sought to understand cause and effect relationships. They believed that if they understood which variables caused social problems (e.g., poverty or crime), they could intervene and "re-engineer" society. They could solve those problems.

Early sociology was premised on the notion that if we could learn the causes of human behavior, we could manipulate those causes to achieve a different (better) outcome. As an example, we could look at criminal behavior and argue that if we knew what variables caused people to commit crimes, we could change those initial conditions and eradicate criminal behavior. Sociologists sought to do this with the use of experiments and surveys. Data were converted into numbers, which they then analyzed using statistics. They believed they could discover "laws" about society the way that natural scientists believed they had discovered laws about things such as gravity and entropy (we know now that many of those natural laws were incorrect, but that's a discussion for another place).

It turns out, though, that social behavior was much more complex than cause and effect relationships. Imagine that instead of a linear relationship between two variables (X → Y), social behavior is a giant spiderweb of interactions, filled with connections, blowing slightly in a breeze. Movement on one strand of the web influences other parts of the web in unpredictable ways. That's a better model of social behavior—one that is non-linear and chaotic. Complexity theorists call this the butterfly effect; small permutations in one part of a system can lead to large, unpredictable changes in another part of the system. A butterfly flapping its wings in Brazil could permutate through the atmospheric system and help create a tornado in Oklahoma.

There are cases in which cause and effect research is the best tool to use—think about John Snow and the Broad Street Pump. Considered the founder of epidemiology, Snow used maps of cases of illness to discover that water from a particular pump in London was contaminated with cholera. When the handle was removed and people could no longer get water from that pump, the outbreak quelled. There are times when health researchers need to find out the cause and effect of an event as a pragmatic concern. As Gullion (2018: 60) writes,

> What caused x disease outbreak is more pragmatic than philosophical during the outbreak itself. Learning that turning off a contaminated water source will stop a cholera outbreak, for example, is obviously an important finding and we don't need much philosophical depth to discover it.

But most of the time, social life is too complex to reduce behavior to simple cause and effect. Although we might not be able to identify cause and effect, we do have the ability to understand more about that spiderweb of social life with qualitative methods. Instead of worrying about cause and effect, we can explore how various components within the system (strands or connections within the spiderweb) operate.

As you work on your own research projects, keep in mind what it is you want to learn when you do research. What is the question that drives your work? From that starting point, you can begin to determine the best ways to find answers to that question.

What is the question that drives your work?

Many students in the health professions say that they've chosen their field of study so that they can go on to make the world a better place. They want to help people, to give people better quality lives. This is a social justice orientation, which also asks researchers to be cautious about techniques that could contribute to silencing or colonizing other groups of people. Some researchers either have chosen to study groups they already are members of or have turned to autoethnography (which we discuss in a later chapter) as a way to protect their research participants from possible exploitation.

Evidence-based methodology (in the form of experiments) has come to be the gold standard for research in medicine and the health sciences. This has influenced how people think social science should be done (Lather 2009). Using this method, researchers conduct experiments to test hypotheses, generally in laboratory settings. Data are quantified, and researchers perform statistical tests to determine whether or not a significant difference exists between cases (people who experienced some sort of intervention as part of the experiment) and controls (people who did not experience the intervention).

Reliability, validity, and objectivity are important components of experimental methods. Reliability is the ability to replicate research. An instrument is said to be reliable if one gets the same results every time it is used. Validity speaks to the soundness and trustworthiness of one's data. We've already discussed objectivity—the idea that neither the researcher nor outside factors should influence the outcome of the research.

The simple example of a bathroom scale is useful for understanding these terms. Suppose a researcher has a ten-pound weight. Every time the researcher puts that weight on the scale, the scale should read ten pounds. If it does, the scale is said to be reliable. The researcher knows the weight is ten pounds, so the scale is said to be valid if the output is ten, as opposed to five or fifteen or some other number. It accurately represents what it is measuring. The scale is thought to be an objective measure because the researcher's feelings and opinions about the weight have no impact on the results that the scale shows.

Underlying evidence-based research is the idea that by providing a control group, the experiment is objective. Denzin (2010: 23) writes that "evidence-based researchers fail to understand that all facts are value- and theory-laden; there is no objective truth." As we will see repeatedly in this text, human behavior is complex and difficult to capture. This does not mean we should discount experimental research—evidence-based methods have generated good knowledge, particularly in the health fields. For example, evidence-based research is used to study the efficacy of drugs or vaccines. It is not as useful for understanding why people don't take their medication or why they won't get vaccinated. While evidence-based research is highly valued, it is not the only way of understanding the world, and it is usually impossible to use to study the types of research questions we seek to answer.

Misconceptions About Qualitative Research

At the start of every semester, I ask my qualitative methods students what assumptions they have heard about qualitative research. Their list of concerns is predictably the same every year. Perhaps you hold some of those concerns as well. Typically, I hear:

1. Qualitative research is less rigorous than quantitative research.
2. Qualitative research is biased and anecdotal.
3. A qualitative dissertation takes longer than a quantitative dissertation.
4. Qualitative research is not publishable.
5. People who do qualitative research can't find jobs.

You might have some of these same concerns. Let's explore each of them.

Qualitative Research Is Less Rigorous Than Quantitative Research

One semester, a student in my methods class said, "I thought qualitative was just loosy-goosy. Like you just did it." She was annoyed that I had asked the class to articulate the philosophical stance they used in their research. It doesn't take students long to figure out that qualitative research is systematic, with a strong basis in theory and contemplative practices. As discussed earlier, systematic qualitative research dates back to the late 1800s—and since then much has been written on how to do social science. Qualitative researchers value transparency in research; that is, good qualitative researchers should specify in their writing exactly what they did to arrive at their conclusions so that the reader can make an informed decision about the usefulness of the research. When done properly, qualitative research is, in fact, quite rigorous. When we conduct research, we create new knowledge. There are codified ways of doing this.

Qualitative Research Is Biased and Anecdotal

We will explore objectivity in more depth, but for now let's talk about bias. To be biased, the researcher would be looking for, even advocating for, a particular outcome. I would venture a guess that many researchers have an idea of what they hope to find as they conduct their research. It is a serious problem, though, when any researcher is blinded to the possibility that they may be wrong. It is a serious ethical problem if they manipulate the data to fit their idea of what the outcome should be. Unfortunately, academic dishonesty occurs in any field of study. Thus, it is not that qualitative research is biased, but it can be the case that the researcher is (whether the study is qualitative, quantitative, experimental, and so forth). Research misconduct happens, and we need to be ethical in our work.

One way to push back against the claim that qualitative research is biased is with a technique called reflexivity. We explore reflexivity in more detail later in this book. For now, let's think of reflexivity as the ways in which the researcher considers how who they are as a person might influence the outcome of their research. Qualitative researchers consider the role that their standpoint—who they are, their experiences, their beliefs—has in the creation of the research as well as in the ways in which they interpret their data. Diffraction is also something that researchers should take into consideration. This is when researchers consider the ways in which they and their participants are both changed by the act of research and the creation of something new together (Gullion 2018).

Anecdote refers to incidents that are quirky or unusual in some way. Arguing that qualitative research is anecdotal and therefore invalid is one way that people try to dismiss this type of inquiry. Qualitative researchers collect and analyze people's stories and their interpretations of their experiences. We believe that people can articulate their own perspective on their own lives (in their own way) and that that is valuable information.

A Qualitative Dissertation Takes Longer Than a Quantitative Dissertation

Let's talk a bit about dissertations (or theses or professional papers—whichever project is called for you to complete your degree). I've served on many dissertation committees, both as chair and as member. I can tell you that there are two predictors that explain how long I've seen it take students to finish and graduate. The first is how intellectually interested they are in their project. The more interested they are, the more likely they are to work on their dissertations and finish. When a researcher is bored with their topic, writing is drudgery and it takes them much longer to do the work. The second predictor of how long it will take them to finish is what's going on in their personal lives. Things happen that get in the way of their research. Students get married, have babies, have health problems, lose loved ones, move, take full-time jobs, and so on. Life simply gets in the way of researching and writing.

Whether the project is qualitative or quantitative doesn't seem to make a difference. It *is* important, however, to work with your committee chair to find a project broad enough in scope to produce a final product worthy of the degree you are seeking and narrow enough that you can realistically complete the work in the usual time allotment.

Qualitative Research Is Not Publishable

In terms of publishing, we should begin with a consideration of the vast array of publication outlets. Although there are arguments over just how many academic journals there are, a generally accepted number is that there are approximately 28,000 reputable journals, with approximately 1.8 million articles published annually (Eveleth 2014). *The Qualitative Report* keeps a list of high-quality journals (curated by Ronald J. Chinaili) that accept qualitative research articles.[2] Note this is not all-inclusive (there are likely journals it has missed), and it only includes English-language journals.

We can also publish in venues other than journals. Academic and trade presses publish books based on qualitative research (look at the fame of Brené Brown; she uses interviews and grounded theory to write her popular, best-selling books). You can also publish in other venues online and in print that may not be peer-reviewed but let you get your findings in the hands of the people who need them. Consider, for example, the vast array of health-related magazines and websites. We will talk more about how to publish in Chapter 10, but know that you have many options when it comes to publishing your work.

Qualitative Researchers Can't Get Jobs

In terms of jobs, while I understand employment is a top concern for students, rest assured that you can find qualitative researchers at pretty much every university. Most degrees in the health professions require that students take at least one research methods course, and the ability to teach those courses will help you get an academic job. I got my job because my department was searching for someone who could teach both qualitative methods and medical sociology. There are also jobs outside of academia in which the skills you learn in qualitative methods courses would be transferable. Indeed, this is most likely the scenario for health practitioners. As you saw earlier, qualitative research methods were invaluable to my work as an epidemiologist.

Ontology and Epistemology, or What Is Real and How Do We Know It's Real?

Now that we've reviewed some of the history and background of qualitative research, let's turn to the philosophy that underlies qualitative inquiry. We begin with a discussion of ontology and epistemology.

Ontology asks: What is a thing? What is reality? Epistemology asks: How do you know the thing is real? How do you understand what is real? These are important questions because your answers reflect the ways in which you understand the world. That understanding then has an impact on your research. Think of philosophy as a lens that you look through to see the world. To extend the metaphor, if my lens is blue and yours is red, we see the world differently. We come to different conclusions about what we see. It's important to be aware of what lenses you use when you conduct research because they influence what and how you see.

Ontology is the study of the nature of reality. A person's perception of what is real colors their vision of the world in a certain way. For example, when I worked in public health, patients often came into the clinic with type II diabetes or metabolic syndrome. The physicians used specific biomedical indicators to define these conditions, along with associated treatments (e.g., dietary changes, exercise, and medication). They did this because of what they believed was real: Diabetes is a biomedical disease. Meanwhile, some of the Mexican immigrants who came into the clinic with what the physician defined as type II diabetes or metabolic syndrome believed that they actually suffered from *susto*—a magical fright in which the soul leaves the body. This fright could have occurred many years ago, but it was manifesting now as this particular health condition. There are regional differences to treating *susto* (Moreira et al. 2018), but the central idea is that to cure the illness one needs to return the missing part of the soul to the body. The two groups—the physicians and the immigrants—perceive reality differently. If the patient believes their condition comes from missing parts of their soul, diet changes and exercise may not make sense to do. This is why cultural humility is so important in medical work. Ideally, the two understandings of reality would work in harmony to heal the patient. Ontology is important because it shapes what we believe is or isn't real and how we respond to that belief.

When approaching research ontologically, we ask, *How does this phenomena work*? This is opposed to asking, *What does this mean*? That question is the realm of epistemology.

Epistemological questions explore knowledge and how people come to know a thing. We ask questions such as what "counts" as knowledge, who gets to make knowledge claims, and why people think the way they do. This also raises questions about how and why people make meaning of phenomena.

Epistemology has a political dimension in that some people can hold epistemic privilege over others (Gullion 2015, 2018). Knowledge-making practices are not neutral: "Knowledge is inherently political and contains a power dimension," Gullion (2018: 13) writes. This is because a person or group holds epistemic privilege when their way of knowing is considered superior to another person's way of knowing. In some cases, this may be appropriate—a cardiologist's understanding of heart disease should be privileged over what I know about it. In other cases, epistemic privilege may be silencing legitimate voices.

In my community, there is a man who drives a car decorated in slogans proclaiming that the Earth is flat. His front lawn is similarly decorated, with signs and information about how to access his YouTube videos on the subject (much to his neighbors' chagrin). I have watched some of his videos out of curiosity. There he makes his epistemic case. He lays out an argument as to how he came to the belief that the Earth is flat. He does not hold epistemic privilege, however. His is a minority perspective, and there is a plethora of scientific evidence that he is wrong.

The gold standard for assigning epistemic privilege is through the use of science. In the flat Earth controversy, science (typically) wins. The Earth is indeed round. The idea that science is the gold standard falls apart, though, when the science is contested.

In my research on natural gas extraction and fracking (Gullion 2015), I found that oil and gas companies had epistemic privilege over people who claimed their health conditions were being caused by natural gas activities. In this case, the science was contested. There are many scientific studies on the health effects of natural gas extraction, some conducted by academics, some by government agencies, and some by the oil and gas companies. But the scientific reports conflict with each other. Research was weaponized, criticized, and discounted based on its methodology.

In the cases of contested knowledge, the people with the most social capital typically hold epistemic privilege, and other ways of knowing are discounted. The oil and gas companies had money and power and attorneys. The residents did not. Gullion (2015: 134) writes that "epistemic privilege is important because public policy is framed and informed by the knowledge that is considered legitimate or 'correct.'"

Gullion (2015: 134–135) continues:

Consider a community embedded in time and space. An object (in this case, natural gas development activities) is inserted into that community. Members of the community then attempt to make sense of that object. They create a representation—a narrative explanation of how the object fits into their social reality. The representation is considered to be social because it emerges through social interaction, through discursive practice, through discussion and counter-discussion, in a variety of textual and geographic spaces. This type of knowledge construction, however, is neither neutral nor democratic—more powerful groups dominate this process and silence less powerful voices.

When one group holds epistemic privilege, minority viewpoints are either discounted or considered to be incorrect. But what if the minority viewpoints are actually correct? Peat (2002: 42) writes that

when Western science claims to be speaking with the truth then, by implication, other people's truths become myths, legends, superstitions, and fairy stories. A dominant society denies the authenticity of other peoples' systems of knowledge and in this way strikes at the very heart of their cultures.

Ontology ⟶ Epistemology ⟶ Methodology

What is real · How we know what is real · The tools we use to measure what is real

FIGURE 1.1 Philosophical basis of research.

As we conduct research, we need to consider what other people think is real (ontology) and how they know things to be true (epistemology). We also need to think about what *we* think is real and how we come to know things, because those ideas will influence our research (Figure 1.1). As Pascale (2011: 3) writes, "All research is anchored to basic beliefs about how the world exists." To get at the heart of what we believe, qualitative researchers practice reflexivity and diffraction. We explore those concepts in more depth later in this book.

Ontology and epistemology form the basis of our measurement tools. We construct our tools to measure various bits and bobs because we believe those bits and bobs are real, that they are things that can be measured. Measurement tools, however, are arbitrary. I can show you how big an inch is, or demonstrate how long a kilometer is, but truly, some human made them up. They were made up because of someone's understanding of the nature of reality, and other people found them useful and adopted them.

Methodology

Methodology refers to the philosophical exploration of the tools we use (e.g., research methods) to understand epistemology and ontology and to create knowledge. Fox and Alldred (2017: 19) write that "all knowledge should be seen as situated. Scientific inquiry is not neutral; every research design, method or theory is an 'agential cut' that reflects a particular power-laden effort to create 'knowledge.'"

Throughout this book, we explore a number of qualitative methods for gathering and analyzing empirical materials (or data). These include in-depth interviewing, participant observation, narrative research, and community-based action research. This is not a comprehensive overview of all possible qualitative methods, but it will give you a strong foundation in the most common ways that qualitative researchers conduct their research.

As you decide on a method for your own research, I recommend that you read more in-depth about that particular method and that you read journal articles and scholarly books in which the author(s) used that method. This way, you can better understand how different researchers use the same method in practice.

Inductive and Deductive Reasoning

Now that we've reviewed some of the philosophy behind conducting inquiry, let's move into some discussion of the nature of scientific research. We begin with a discussion of inductive and deductive reasoning.

Most likely, you learned how to do science at a young age. You were presented with the following model: To do science, one begins with a theory, writes hypotheses to test that theory, conducts an experiment to gather data that will be used to either support or not

TABLE 1.1 Types of Reasoning

Deductive Reasoning	Inductive Reasoning
Begins with theory	Begins with observations
Derives hypotheses to test the theory	Analyzes the data
Collects data to support or not support the hypotheses	Looks for patterns or concepts
Analyzes the data	Tests patterns or concepts
Refines the theory	Writes a new theory

support the hypotheses, and, finally, presents the results. This is called the scientific method, or positivistic research, and involves deductive reasoning. In most cases, the data are quantitative (i.e., represented by numbers), and validity and reliability are important markers of how well the researcher performed the science. Validity may be defined as how well the instrument used represents reality, and reliability refers to getting the same results every time the instrument is used.

Inductive reasoning works backward from deductive reasoning. Inductive reasoning begins with gathering observations about a phenomena of interest. The researcher then analyzes the data, searching for themes or patterns or concepts in the data. Once those have been identified, the researcher goes back through the data to see if that finding persists across the data. If it does, then the researcher writes a theory.

Qualitative research can be inductive or deductive, although qualitative researchers typically use inductive reasoning. Which you use depends on how you set up your study (Table 1.1).

Examples of deductive methods include experiments, survey research, and demographic research. Examples of inductive methods include in-depth interviewing, ethnography, and focus groups. It is sometimes the case that people partaking in a population-based survey are invited to do an in-depth interview after they have completed the survey. This type of mixed method approach is common. Likewise, researchers can take information they discovered in in-depth interviews and use it to build surveys for population-based research. Using mixed approaches, the researcher draws on both inductive and deductive reasoning. Using multiple techniques allows the researcher to triangulate, or confirm, their findings. Mixed methods are also used for breadth—with the population-based methods—and depth—with intense one-on-one interaction with some of the participants about the subject of the survey.

Whether we use inductive or deductive reasoning can be influenced by our use of theory, so let's discuss theory next.

Theory

I have found that research and theory are often taught as if they are separable, and as a result, students have difficulty integrating the two (Figure 1.2). They come up with an idea

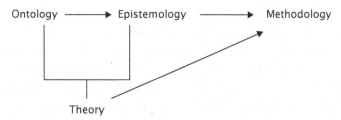

FIGURE 1.2 Theory in philosophical orientation.

they are interested in and then go back to find a theory that seems to fit their idea. Although this is certainly one way to do research, it is backward from how science is supposed to be done (this is also different from grounded theory, which we explore in Chapter 9).

> Theories are systems of ideas intended to explain a phenomena.

Theories are systems of ideas intended to explain a phenomenon. We use them to guide our own thinking. If we approach a problem with a feminist orientation, we will probably ask different questions and look at data differently than if we approach a problem from a symbolic interactionist perspective. For example, let's consider people who refuse to get the COVID-19 vaccine, despite the global pandemic. Looking at this through a feminist lens, we might ask questions about the power dynamics involved with this group. We could consider the conflict between people who received the vaccine and those who refuse to be vaccinated, and who benefits at whose expense. If, instead, we considered this issue from a symbolic interactionist lens, we might ask what the vaccine means to people, what it represents. We might ask, What does refusing the vaccine mean to people? What does getting the vaccine represent? How do the meanings of the vaccine configure group identity?

Theory and theorizing about the subject of our research are what differentiate social scientists from journalists. We do more than report on events; we analyze them using a particular theoretical perspective. We do this whether we realize it or not. We all have our own lens, our own standpoint, that comes from our experiences and identities. We use this lens every day to interpret the world. If, in doing research, we are not explicit about our theoretical orientation, we are in danger of introducing bias into our analysis.

One of the best discussions I have found on how to use theory in qualitative research is Jackson and Mazzei's book, *Thinking with Theory in Qualitative Research* (2012). In their text, the authors demonstrate how to fold theory and data intra-actively into each other, to gain insights both into the data and into the theory. "Data," they write, "are partial, incomplete, and always in a process of a re-telling and re-membering" (ix). Because of this, we use theory as a lens through which to look at the stories we collect. Jackson and Mazzei push us to use theory as a means to deterritorialize (in a Deluezian sense) boundaries and open new possibilities for building knowledge.

Rather than focus on individuals, Jackson and Mazzei (2012) advocate for a focus on events and phenomena. We talk more about unit of analysis in Chapter 3, but for now, we define it as the thing or entity under investigation. We then investigate the entity as if the theorist we are using to guide our thinking is sitting next to us. Based on the theorist's writings, what would the theorist ask about this entity? How would they interpret what the entity is doing, what is happening to the entity, how the entity intra-acts in the world? Latour (2005: 47) writes that "every single interview, narrative, and commentary, no matter how trivial it may appear, will provide the analyst with a bewildering array of entities to account for the hows and whys of any course of action." This reinforces the importance of having an analytical lens with which to conduct our inquiry.

Gaukroger (2012: 41) writes,

> The world itself presents itself to us as a flux of impressions which have little coherence in their own right. It is the task of the mind to organize these impressions into discrete ingredients, connect these by way of concepts, and ascribe significance to various parts of the world as perceived.

Theory is a tool that helps us do this in a systematic, rigorous way.

When we think with theory, we cannot force data to fit our theory. Rather, our data may tell us there's a problem with the theory. Thinking with theory is an organic process, an iterative folding and flattening origami. The theory informs understanding of the phenomena, while the phenomena inform the theory.

Sometimes it can feel like qualitative researchers are not that different from journalists—we report on the things people do and say and feel. Although there are times when we want to do journalistic work, we move beyond journalism when we engage in theoretical and interpretive work.

Unless you are conducting grounded theory and using qualitative methods to write your own theory (which we discuss later), your work should be informed by theory. Social scientists have a large body of theory to work with, with many different scholars and lineages to choose from, and you should be well-versed in the theories used in your particular field. Read all of the theory you can in order to understand which best informs your research. Theory should be your starting point and not a section that is tacked on to your manuscript after the fact.

Deciding which theory you would like to think with can be a bit overwhelming. It's important that you read widely to get a sense of whose work resonates with you. Although there are more theorists than I could possibly list here, there are general schools of thought that you might wish to explore. I touch on some of them here, but an in-depth discussion of theorists within these schools is beyond the scope of this book.

We begin with positivism and post-positivism because those are the most familiar to people. Positivists believe there is an external reality "out there" that is measurable. They use theory to generate testable hypotheses to support (or not support) the original theory. If the data do not support the theory, they consider whether or not the theory should be refined.

Critical theory encompasses feminism, race, postcolonial, transnational, endarkened, queer, disabilities, and other identity theorists who delve into social problems in order to critique them and to push for social change. Critical race theory (CRT), in particular, has come under attack in the United States by social conservatives who don't like what CRT uncovers about institutional racism and the ongoing legacy of slavery. Critical theorists have a social justice orientation and are interested in power—who has it, who doesn't, and how power is used to abuse and exploit people.

Symbolic interactionists, structuralists, and post-structuralists look at language, discourse, and signs, albeit in different ways. This area of theorizing is interested in meaning and meaning-making activities.

Constructionists explore the ways in which people construct the social world, build a collective consciousness and shared realities, through material and discursive practices.

New materialists, posthumanists, and object-oriented ontologists consider the ways in which the human and nonhuman intra-act. They dismantle ontological hierarchies and consider the agencies of nonhuman actors, including objects.

This is a very small glimpse into possibilities for how to frame your study with theory. Read as much theory as you can so that you can develop a sense of what paradigm you would like to work from.

Decolonizing Research

I'd like for us to turn now to different debates and discourses current within the field of qualitative methodology. I want you to be aware of these conversations so that you know how to address them in your own work and so that you can respond to questions that you might be asked as you put your work out into the world. We begin with a look at decolonizing research. Smith (2012: 8) writes that

> research is one of the ways in which the underlying code of imperialism and colonialism is both regulated and realized. It is regulated through the formal rules of individual scholarly disciplines and scientific paradigms, and the institutions that support them (including the state). It is realized in the myriad of representations and ideological constructions of the Other in scholarly and "popular" works, and in the principles which help to select and recontextualize those constructions in such things as the media, official histories and school curricula.

There is a history of *othering* in social science research. One group of people (historically, White males) is held as the "standard" against which other groups are compared. A Western, Enlightenment-informed perspective is often used in which "outsiders" are positioned as "exotic" or "deficient." A significant body of current social science literature is concerned with comparing groups and looking for statistical differences and similarities between them. Often in statistical tests, Whites are held as the reference group to which Peoples of Color are compared.

As an example, we might think about studies on infant mortality rates, in which Whites are compared to Blacks. While it might not be explicit in the document, there is an underlying assumption that because Black infant mortality is greater than White infant mortality, Black mothers are to blame for not keeping their babies alive. That is a terrible way in which Black women are othered. What if instead we looked at racism in access to and delivery of health care, shifting the "blame" to the system, taking it to task to eliminate this disparity? In this case, mothers are not to blame—internalized, systematic racism within the health care system is.

Canons of intellectual thought are dominated by the writings of White men. For too long, White men were the only ones with access to higher education and to publishing venues. Although that is changing, the intellectual contribution of a fairly homogeneous population of scholars is a legacy we still engage. Scheurich (2018: 126) writes,

> If you mix in the fact that university social science researchers are overwhelmingly visually white, financially upper middle class, evidently male, apparently heterosexual, temporarily able, and fundamentally Christian and highly influenced by the dominant narrative, and its privileging of these positionalities, you get a very potent and toxic mix. You get a contemporary version of a colonizer, a very small, a very powerful elite who individually are naming and constructing the social "reality" in which everyone must live.

Likewise, what "counts" as research has historically been held in narrow confines, shaped by Western philosophy (Bhattacharya and Kim 2018). In other words, knowledge has historically been considered legitimate only when published by White (male) scholars. This does not mean that outside thought does not influence Western thinkers. According to Gullion (2018: 22–23), "Indigenous knowledge systems have been covertly appropriated while they [Indigenous peoples] have simultaneously been systematically excluded." Part of colonization includes absorbing Indigenous philosophy and retooling it as the colonizer's own.

Indigenous knowledge has been appropriated and twisted to become the knowledge of settler–colonialists. We can look at herbal medicine as a good example of this. Herbal medicine has been appropriated by companies selling herbs for their health benefits (or adding them to supplements and food and drinks). Pharmaceutical companies will take the knowledge about the health effects of herbs and break herbal remedies into their constituent parts, to be used proprietarily in making medicines (e.g., the transmutation of willow bark into aspirin) for great financial gain. Meanwhile, Indigenous lands are raped of their plant life, and many wild medicinal herbs are in danger of overharvesting.

Indigenous peoples themselves have been some of the most researched (Smith 2005: 87; Gaudry 2011; Rix et al. 2018). They have been othered in their own lands, and research has been used as justification for their oppression (think here of studies that argue some groups are genetically inferior to others, or the use of social science in warfare). Research has been one tool of colonizers to marginalize Indigenous peoples and other less powerful social groups.

Likewise, research is one means for the reproduction and ongoing telling of colonial narratives. "Narratives of conquest are present, pervasive, and mostly invisible within the settler consciousness," Rowe and Tuck (2016: 4) write,

> yet they are doing profound cultural work in reminding settlers that they belong, that their place in the social order has been hard-won through the taming of the

savages, and confirming their status as the rightful inheritors of pastoral landscapes such scenes evoke.

To decolonize your own research, critically look at your study and see if you are othering a less powerful group of people. Look also at the authors you cite and be sure that you are citing a diverse group of scholars. Attribute knowledge to the correct source.

Sacred Knowledge

Some knowledge is sacred. It is not intended to be shared with outsiders. A Western cultural framework holds that the job of the social scientist is to uncover/discover knowledge. It is difficult to consider that not all knowledge is there for us to consume.

In 2018, members of the Sentinelese tribe in India shot and killed an American man with arrows after he continually tried to encroach onto their protected lands (Pandey 2018). The Sentinelese are a small Indigenous tribe who choose not to interact with outsiders. The Indian government has made it illegal to interact with members of the tribe out of fear that people will unwittingly carry diseases into their community. But this American man decided that he would bring Christianity to them. In fact, this was not his first attempt to do so; he was shot at during previous attempts. Missionaries are often leaders in colonization, and here was this American man, so arrogant to believe that he deserved entrance, that he deserved to know all that these people knew, and then change what they believed.

We cannot go into research with the idea that we *deserve* to know a thing. To have someone give you their knowledge must be treated as an honor, as a gift, not as a right.

Keeping some knowledge hidden is one way people resist the Western knowledge juggernaut. If someone doesn't want to talk with you, *that is their right*. Respect it. If a group does not want you to have knowledge of its sacred practices, respect that and walk away.

Researching Down, Researching Up

Another way that people are othered has to do with the relative power of the researcher to that of the participant. Historically, social science researchers have been preoccupied with the concerns of people with less social capital than they have. Bourdieu (1983: 249) defined social capital as "the aggregate of the actual or potential resources which are linked to possession of a durable network of more or less institutionalized relationships of mutual acquaintance and recognition." In other words, the connections one has to others matter in order to thrive economically in society. People with less social capital are often framed as problematic and pathologic. Meanwhile, people with more social capital are not viewed with the same lens of deviance, even though we know there are great social problems associated with the inequitable division of wealth.

Let's consider prescription opioid addiction as an example. Suppose we have a patient, John, who is seen in an emergency room following a motorcycle accident. He has severe injuries and is given hydrocodone for pain. He is discharged from the emergency room with a thirty-day supply of the drug. John does not have a primary care physician, but after his accident, he finds one. He complains about ongoing pain and is given another thirty-day supply of hydrocodone. While John recovers, he continues to take the medication. When he tries to stop the medication, he develops severe withdrawal symptoms. He goes to an acute care clinic, tells them about the accident, and the physician there gives him a thirty-day supply of hydrocodone. He begins to worry about the possibility of being without the medication, so to be safe, he goes to a different acute care clinic and gets yet another prescription. He fills them at different pharmacies. John has begun drug-seeking behavior; his injuries have healed.

There are two different ways to tackle this example. One would be to say that the patient is at fault—that the patient is a drug addict who has learned how to manipulate the system. The other way to approach this is to look at the structures of power and ask what systems are in place that have allowed John to become an addict. Where is the pathology? Is it in John—who initially was injured and did require pain management—the physicians who prescribe this medication without a plan in place to wean him off of it, or pharmaceutical companies that push opioid sales? Often, researchers would focus on John, the person with the least social capital in this situation. It is easier to ask John for an interview and talk to him about opioids than it is to interview pharmaceutical executives about drug research and development, costs and price points, income ratios, and returns on investments. It is easier to survey John and others like him than to talk with physicians about what (if any) follow-up care they provide after prescribing opioids. Researchers have greater access to people with less social capital than we do primarily because of our own level of social capital. Likewise, we have less access to people who have more social capital than we do.

But good science doesn't come easy. We shouldn't sacrifice knowledge production for what is easier. As Gullion and Tilton (2020: 54) write,

> We need to recognize that while the community group we are researching may have a problem, *they are not the problem*. They are not damaged. They do not need fixing. Rather, we need to explore power and barriers to understand the underlying dynamics of the problem.

Objectivity

I previously mentioned objectivity, and I return to the concept in more depth because it tends to come up often when discussing qualitative research. Objectivity is an important consideration in science, and researchers strive to be objective in the course of their work. To be objective is to keep the researcher from influencing the outcomes of the research. A common criticism of qualitative research is that it is not objective.

To address this criticism, let's think about where this idea originated. Objectivity as a value in knowledge-making practices comes to us from the Enlightenment and positivism.

Students generally tend to come to qualitative research with a background rooted in Enlightenment ideals. From elementary school, they've learned that science looks a certain way: theories with testable hypotheses. They are taught that science involves a knowing subject (the researcher) who studies a passive object. They are taught that numbers (math and science) are more important than words (literature and the arts), that STEM (science, technology, engineering, and mathematics) is more valued than the arts and humanities.

As we become more knowledgeable about the world, we are learning that there are no passive objects. Even items we perceive as solid are active at the molecular (or at the quantum) level. Nonetheless, this fact often remains unacknowledged, or it is glossed over in the business of doing science. Likewise, it is possible that it is not until they reach their first qualitative methods class (sometimes not until graduate school) that students hear that science can look different—or even that "science" may not be the goal at all.

Objectivity is often conflated with quantification. They are not the same thing, yet every time I teach qualitative methods, a student will inevitably argue that qualitative methods are not objective, whereas quantitative methods are.

> Objectivity is often conflated with quantification. They are not the same thing.

When we dig deeper into this argument, we find that rather than worry about qualitative methods, the trouble is that people trust numbers. Some people may argue that qualitative research is not objective because it involves human intervention. A researcher intra-acts with other humans, and the researcher might have an underlying agenda that skews the research findings. That qualitative research is anecdotal rather than quantified. Yet in quantitative research, anecdotes are converted into numbers all the time. Once they are, they become valued. For example, let's return to our patient, John, who was in a motorcycle accident. Suppose we ask him about his pain and he says, "I hurt all the time. It's hard for me to sit for more than half an hour. I have to stand or lie down. It's causing me trouble at work because I have a desk job; I'm supposed to sit all day." This is anecdotal evidence about John's pain. Now the health care worker has to decide how accurate his story is, how debilitating his pain *really* is, and whether or not he is even telling the truth. Now let's suppose a researcher is conducting a population-based survey about living with pain. John is selected to participate. The researcher emails him a link to an online survey that includes questions such as, "On a scale from 1–5 (1 being not at all, 5 being the worst), how bad is your pain?" Now the pain has become a number. Once all of the surveys are collected, the researcher analyzes the data with statistics. The researcher learns that 24 percent of the people in the study have an average pain score of 3.5, and 5 percent have a high average pain score. This is then presented as fact in a journal article: 24 percent of Americans live with pain, and 5 percent of Americans live with high levels of pain.

How much pain is John in? It is a 3? A 5? What do those numbers even mean? At what point does his treatment plan change based on his reported level of pain? While the numbers are treated as reality, they are arbitrary. What is the quantifiable difference between a pain score of 3 or 4? Four or 5?

We might conceptualize objectivity as removing one's preconceptions about what the findings of the project might be. Yet Gaukroger (2012: 37–38) writes, "We cannot perceive or think without assumptions of various kinds, but the fact that there is a grey area between reasonable assumptions and prejudice does not mean that we cannot think without prejudices." And as Marker (2009: 39) notes, "There *is* no disinterested academic." We do the research we do because of our interest in the topics involved.

Which "story" of John's pain do you believe? His anecdote or the number he circled on the survey?

Laboratory sciences, with their case–control studies, are often held as the gold standard of disinterested research. Yet, the question of objectivity is held in those fields as well. Peat (2002: 246) writes that "being an experimenter is closer to being a master chef than to a mechanic or dispassionate computer." When conducting an experiment, the researcher makes many choices involving the parameters and conditions, about how data are created and what empirical materials are important. Things such as the humidity in the room or the level of the lighting can be a problem with some experiments. Peat (2002: 246) writes,

> The very basis of science, its objective, repeatable, quantitative observations and experiments, is an unattainable ideal, for the way scientists are able to design experiments and carry them out is influenced in so many subtle ways by their feelings and sensitivity to the complex world around them.

In other words, *all* research grapples with objectivity. As humans living in the world we study, pure objectivity is impossible.

Another issue to consider is the Hawthorne effect. In the 1920s, workers at the Hawthorne Western Electric plant were subjected to a research study on how lighting impacted their productivity. Researchers found that the subjects changed their behavior because they knew they were being studied and that the researchers were looking for an increase in their productivity. Landsberger (1957) later coined the term Hawthorne effect to describe this phenomenon. Sometimes participants will act differently because of the presence of the researcher, often trying to "give" the researcher what they think the researcher is looking for. They might change their responses to give what they believe are socially acceptable answers (e.g., a person might reduce the reported number of sexual partners they've had out of embarrassment). When this happens, the researcher is not getting an objective understanding of the phenomenon due to the reactions of the participants to the study itself.

What if we reconsidered our enamor of objectivity? Gaukroger (2012: 64) suggests we think about objectivity as the "elimination of arbitrary judgements." This is different from defining objectivity as freedom from human thought/intervention.

Rather than worry about objectivity, many qualitative researchers aim for co-constructed knowledge or a diffractive approach. They recognize that together with the participant knowledge is created and that both parties are changed by their interaction. Knowing that we have an influence on the research process at all stages, they use that as an advantage. The products of research are thus the result of intersections and interactions with participants.

This brings us back to the importance of ontology. Does a Truth (with a capital T) exist outside of humans that we can measure? Or is the world made up of small truths, different truths, truths that are emergent rather than fixed? Also, if a statement is not objective, does that mean it is false?

Notes

1. https://archive.org/details/notesandqueries00readgoog.
2. https://tqr.nova.edu/journals.

References

Atkinson, Paul, Amanda Coffey, Sara Delemont, John Lofland, and Lyn Lofland. 2001. *Handbook of Ethnography*. Los Angeles: SAGE.

Bhattacharya, Kakali, and Jeong-Hee Kim. 2018. "Reworking Prejudice in Qualitative Inquiry with Gadamer and De/Colonizing Onto-Epistemologies." *Qualitative Inquiry* 24, no. 3: 1–10.

Bourdieu, Pierre. 1983. "Forms of Capital." In *Handbook of Theory and Research for the Sociology of Education*, edited by John G. Richardson, 241–258. New York: Greenwood.

Deegan, Mary Jo. 2001. "The Chicago School of Ethnography." In *Handbook of Ethnography*, edited by Paul Atkinson, Amanda Coffey, Sara Delamont, John Lofland, and Lyn Lofland, 11–25. London: SAGE.

Denzin, Norman. K. 2010. *The Qualitative Manifesto: A Call to Arms*. Walnut Creek, CA: Left Coast Press.

DuBois, W. E. B. 1899. *The Philadelphia Negro: A Social Study*. Philadelphia: University of Pennsylvania Press.

Erickson, Frederick. 2018. "A History of Qualitative Inquiry in Social Science and Educational Research." In *The SAGE Handbook of Qualitative Research*, 5th ed., edited by Norman K. Denzin and Yvonna S. Lincoln, 36–65. Los Angeles: SAGE.

Eveleth, Rose. 2014. "Academic Write Papers Arguing Over How Many People Read (and Cite) Their Papers." *Smithsonian Magazine*. Accessed January 31, 2020. https://www.smithsonianmag.com/smart-news/half-academic-studies-are-never-read-more-three-people-180950222.

Fox, Nick J., and Pam Alldred. 2017. *Sociology and the New Materialism: Theory, Research, Action*. Los Angeles: SAGE.

Gane, Nicholas. 2011. "Measure, Value, and the Current Crisis in Sociology." *Sociological Review* 59, no. 2: 151–173.

Gaudry, Adam J. 2011. "Insurgent Research." *Wicazo Sa Review* 26, no. 1: 113–136.

Gaukroger, Stephen. 2012. *Objectivity: A Very Short Introduction*. New York: Oxford University Press.

Gullion, Jessica Smartt. 2015. *Fracking the Neighborhood: Reluctant Activists and Natural Gas Drilling*. Cambridge, MA: MIT Press.

Gullion, Jessica Smartt. 2018. *Diffractive Ethnography: Social Sciences in the Ontological Turn*. London: Routledge.

Gullion, Jessica Smartt, and Abigail Tilton. 2020. *Researching With: A Decolonizing Approach to Community-Based Action Research*. Rotterdam, the Netherlands: Brill/Sense.

Jackson, Alecia Y., and Lisa A. Mazzei. 2012. *Thinking with Theory in Qualitative Research: Viewing Data Across Multiple Perspectives*. New York: Routledge.

King, Charles. 2019. *Gods of the Upper Air: How a Circle of Renegade Anthropologists Reinvented Race, Sex, and Gender in the Twentieth Century*. New York: Doubleday.

Landsberger, Henry A. 1957. *Hawthorne Revisited: A Plea for an Open City*. Ithaca, NY: Cornell University Press.

Lather, Patti. 2009. *Engaging Science Policy: From the Side of the Messy*. New York: Lang.

Latour, Bruno. 2005. *Reassembling the Social: An Introduction to Actor-Network-Theory*. Oxford, UK: Oxford University Press.

MacDonald, Sharon. 2001. "British Social Anthropology." In *Handbook of Ethnography*, edited by Paul Atkinson, Amanda Coffey, Sara Delamont, John Lofland, and Lyn Lofland, 60–79. Los Angeles: SAGE.

Malinowski, Bronislaw. 1922/2016. *Argonauts of the Western Pacific: An Account of Native Enterprise and Adventure in the Archipelagos of Melanesia New Guinea*. London: Oxford University Press.

Marker, Michael. 2009. "Indigenous Voice, Community, and Epistemic Violence: The Ethnographer's 'Interests' and What 'Interests' the Ethnographer." In *Voice in Qualitative Inquiry: Challenging Conventional, Interpretive, and Critical Conceptions in Qualitative Research*, edited by A. Y. Jackson and L. A. Mazzei, 27–43. New York: Routledge.

Maynes, Mary Jo, Jennifer L. Piece, and Barbara Laslett. 2008. *Telling Stories: The Use of Personal Narratives in the Social Sciences and History*. Ithaca, NY: Cornell University Press.

Moreira, Telma, Daphne C. Hernandez, Claudia W. Scott, Rosenda Murillo, Elizabeth M. Vaughan, and Craig A. Johnston. 2018. *"Susto, Coraje, y Fatalismo*: Cultural-Bound Beliefs and the Treatment of Diabetes Among Socioeconomically Disadvantaged Hispanics." *American Journal of Lifestyle Medicine* 12, no. 1: 30–33.

Pandey, Geeta. 2018. "American Killed in India by Endangered Andamans Tribe." BBC News. Accessed November 2018. https://www.bbc.com/news/world-asia-india-46286215.

Pascale, Celine-Marie. 2011. *Cartographies of Knowledge: Exploring Qualitative Epistemologies*. London: SAGE.

Peat, F. David, 2002. *Blackfoot Physics*. Boston: Red Wheel/Weiser.

Rix, Elizabeth F., Shawn Wilson, Norm Sheehan, and Nicole Tujague. 2018. "Indigenist and Decolonizing Research Methodology." In *Handbook of Research Methods in Health Social Sciences*, edited by Pranee Liamputtong, 1–15. Singapore: Springer.

Rowe, Aimee Carrillo, and Eve Tuck. 2016. "Settler Colonialism and Cultural Studies: Ongoing Settlement, Cultural Production, and Resistance." *Cultural Studies ↔ Critical Methodologies* 17, no. 1: 1–11.

Scheurich, James Joseph. 2018. "Research 4 Revolutionaries by #Jimscheurish." In *Qualitative Inquiry in the Public Sphere*, edited by Norman K. Denzin and Michael D. Giardina, 125–142. New York: Routledge.

Smith, Linda Tuhiwai. 2005. "On Tricky Ground: Researching the Native in the Age of Uncertainty." In *The SAGE Handbook of Qualitative Research*, 4th ed., edited by Norman K. Denzin and Yvonna S. Lincoln, 85–107. Thousand Oaks, CA: SAGE.

Smith, Linda Tuhiwai. 2012. *Decolonizing Methodologies: Research and Indigenous Peoples*, 2nd ed. New York: Zed Books.

FURTHER READING

Denzin, Norman K. 2010. *The Qualitative Manifesto: A Call to Arms*. Walnut Creek, CA: Left Coast Press.

King, Charles. 2019. *Gods of the Upper Air: How a Circle of Renegade Anthropologists Reinvented Race, Sex, and Gender in the Twentieth Century*. New York: Doubleday.

Lather, Patti. 2009. *Engaging Science Policy: From the Side of the Messy*. New York: Lang.

Discussion Questions

1. Have you ever conducted qualitative research or been part of a qualitative research project? Describe that experience.
2. Why should we decolonize our research? How can we go about doing that?
3. What theories of health and illness resonate with you? How might they help you conduct research?

Active Learning

1. Talk to faculty members in your department about the research methods that they use and why they use them. Determine if there are any allegiances to particular methods and why those exist.
2. Search for peer-reviewed journals that publish qualitative research. Read articles related to your research interests.

Mindfulness Exercises

1. What is reality? How do you determine what is real?
2. If experience, time, and money were not barriers, and you could research anything you wanted to, what would you choose? Why?

2

Research Ethics

In this chapter, we explore ethical issues related to research. This includes legal considerations, historical abuses, the standards for ethical research, mitigation of risks to participants, and working with special populations. We also look closely at the role and work
of institutional review boards and consider their scope. Finally, we examine different
types of ethical considerations, including procedural, situational, and relational ethics.

Although extraordinary good can come from social and behavioral research, anytime we
work with other people, the potential exists for their mistreatment. In this chapter, we explore the history of ethical protections for human subjects research (i.e., any research on
or about people). We also discuss current legislation on ethical research practices and how
to mitigate ethical problems in your own work. It is important to note that most of the
information in this chapter comes from U.S. law. Although still relevant internationally,
researchers working outside of the United States should familiarize themselves with the
specific rules that apply to them. It is also important to note from the start that we must be
mindful of research ethics *throughout* our projects. Ethics is not a one-time consideration
but, rather, should be a concern from inception to completion of your research.

We must be mindful of ethics throughout the research process—from start to finish.

We begin by conceptu-
alizing some of the terms we
will use in this discussion. The
first is the term "research." The
U.S. federal definition of research is narrow and does not
always align with how academics colloquially use the term. Much of the scholarly activity
in the humanities and the arts is not considered research under federal guidelines, but it is
certainly considered research by faculty in those fields. In addition, some types of qualitative research do not meet the federal definition of research.

Qualitative Research in Health and Illness. Jessica Smartt Gullion, Oxford University Press. © Oxford University Press 2024.
DOI: 10.1093/oso/9780190915988.003.0003

The Federal Policy for the Protection of Human Subjects (National Archives and Records Administration, 2018), also known as the Common Rule, defines research as such:

> *Research* means a systematic investigation, including research development, testing, and evaluation, designed to develop or contribute to generalizable knowledge. Activities that meet this definition constitute research for purposes of this policy, whether or not they are conducted or supported under a program that is considered research for other purposes. For example, some demonstration and service programs may include research activities. For purposes of this part, the following activities are deemed not to be research:
>
> 1. Scholarly and journalistic activities (e.g., oral history, journalism, biography, literary criticism, legal research, and historical scholarship), including the collection and use of information, that focus directly on the specific individuals about whom the information is collected.
> 2. Public health surveillance activities, including the collection and testing of information or biospecimens, conducted, supported, requested, ordered, required, or authorized by a public health authority. Such activities are limited to those necessary to allow a public health authority to identify, monitor, assess, or investigate potential public health signals, onsets of disease outbreaks, or conditions of public health importance (including trends, signals, risk factors, patterns in diseases, or increases in injuries from using consumer products). Such activities include those associated with providing timely situational awareness and priority setting during the course of an event or crisis that threatens public health (including natural or man-made disasters).
> 3. Collection and analysis of information, biospecimens, or records by or for a criminal justice agency for activities authorized by law or court order solely for criminal justice or criminal investigative purposes.
> 4. Authorized operational activities (as determined by each agency) in support of intelligence, homeland security, defense, or other national security missions.

We also want to conceptualize what we mean by "human subjects." For this, the Common Rule states,

> 1. *Human subject* means a living individual about whom an investigator (whether professional or student) conducting research:
>   i. Obtains information or biospecimens through intervention or interaction with the individual, and uses, studies, or analyzes the information or biospecimens; or
>   ii. Obtains, uses, studies, analyzes, or generates identifiable private information or identifiable biospecimens.

When defining what it means to be a human subject, the first criteria is that we are talking about living persons. Research on dead people does not fall under human subjects protection, although other legislation and disciplinary ethical codes may speak to the protection of privacy after death.

The second criteria is that we are talking about research on people as persons, their behavior, personal characteristics, opinions, and so forth. Social scientists may tread in some murky waters here—some questions you might ask may not fall under this definition. For example, if I ask a health care provider how many patients her clinic sees per day, I am not asking about her specifically, and that question falls outside this rule.

Next, we want to consider our interventions and interactions with the participants, with the humans in our study. An intervention might include a physical act, gathering biomedical specimens, for example, or an intervention could be behavioral, such as having participants go through a training program and evaluating the effectiveness of it with a pre- and post-test. Similarly, we can have interactions with the participant during which we collect information. This could be something like a survey or focus group. Interactions do not have to be face-to-face; we can interact with them online or remotely as well. In any case, we are interfering with the subject in some manner and collecting information about and during that interference.

There are many scholarly activities that involve human subjects but are not considered research under the federal guidelines. These activities fall outside of the Common Rule. Examples include the following:

- Biography
- Historical research
- Homeland security investigations
- Journalism
- Law enforcement investigations
- Legal research
- Literary criticism
- Oral history
- Public health surveillance

This does not mean that people doing these types of activities can act without regard to ethical behavior—they have disciplinary codes of ethics they are supposed to follow. It simply means that they do not fall under the Common Rule.

Any study that meets the federal definitions of both research and human subjects must be reviewed for ethical compliance by an institution's institutional review board (IRB). We'll talk more about IRBs in a bit, but I want to state here that *if you are ever unclear about whether or not your study falls under the Common Rule, you should speak with your institution's IRB and get documentation of how it defines your work.*

Research is federally defined as a systematic investigation meant to create generalizable knowledge. The work of qualitative researchers is almost never

In the United States, research is federally defined as a systematic investigation meant to create generalizable knowledge.

generalizable, however. To be generalizable, one needs to take a random sample of a defined population, of which every member has an equal chance of selection. This is where qualitative inquiry and federal definitions of research have the potential to get fuzzy. Whereas quantitative research strives to be systematic and statistically generalizable, some qualitative research is not systematic at all, and most of it is not intended to be generalizable. Qualitative researchers often rely on convenience or targeted sampling, which is not generalizable to a larger population.

Unfortunately, the Common Rule does not define the terms systematic or generalizable. In terms of ethical oversight, it is better for us to define both systematic and generalizable broadly and consider whether or not the information obtained in a qualitative study could contribute to a larger body of work on the topic. It is always better for us to err on the side of human subjects protection rather than assume this does not apply to our type of inquiry.

Historical Perspectives

History is ripe with examples of unethical research practices, but we begin with World War II. Nazi medical experiments are notorious for the atrocities committed on concentration camp prisoners. Physicians performed all sorts of horrific tests and procedures on prisoners, without any consent to do so. Their primary rationalization was that data from these experiments could be used to support their military in the war effort. The United States Holocaust Memorial Museum (2006) reports that these experiments fell into three areas:

1. Tests on the ability of soldiers to survive under a variety of conditions
2. Testing of drugs and medical procedures
3. Other tests that would advance the Nazi eugenics platform

Survival experiments included forced high-altitude parachute jumps, freezing people to design treatments for hypothermia, and forcing prisoners to drink seawater to determine how much salinity one could survive drinking. Medical research included experimental bone grafting and other surgical techniques, exposure to chemical compounds for weapons use, and the testing of a wide variety of new drugs. Many prisoners were also forcibly sterilized in the name of eugenics.

In the aftermath of World War II, the Allied countries held trails in Nuremberg, Germany, to bring top-level Nazi war criminals to justice. One of these trials (known as the Doctors' Trial) was specifically for physicians, who were charged with crimes against humanity. What is now known as the Nuremberg Code was drafted during this trial and since has been the foundation for ethical research on human beings.[1]

The Code set standards for informed consent and the ethical treatment of research subjects.

The Nuremberg Code

1. The voluntary consent of the human subject is absolutely essential. This means that the person involved should have legal capacity to give consent; should be so situated as to be able to exercise free power of choice, without the intervention of any element of force, fraud, deceit, duress, over-reaching, or other ulterior form of constraint or coercion; and should have sufficient knowledge and comprehension of the elements of the subject matter involved, as to enable him to make an understanding and enlightened decision. This latter element requires that, before the acceptance of an affirmative decision by the experimental subject, there should be made known to him the nature, duration, and purpose of the experiment; the method and means by which it is to be conducted; all inconveniences and hazards reasonably to be expected; and the effects upon his health or person, which may possibly come from his participation in the experiment. The duty and responsibility for ascertaining the quality of the consent rests upon each individual who initiates, directs or engages in the experiment. It is a personal duty and responsibility which may not be delegated to another with impunity.

2. The experiment should be such as to yield fruitful results for the good of society, unprocurable by other methods or means of study, and not random and unnecessary in nature.

3. The experiment should be so designed and based on the results of animal experimentation and a knowledge of the natural history of the disease or other problem under study, that the anticipated results will justify the performance of the experiment.

4. The experiment should be so conducted as to avoid all unnecessary physical and mental suffering and injury.

5. No experiment should be conducted, where there is an a priori reason to believe that death or disabling injury will occur; except, perhaps, in those experiments where the experimental physicians also serve as subjects.

6. The degree of risk to be taken should never exceed that determined by the humanitarian importance of the problem to be solved by the experiment.

7. Proper preparations should be made and adequate facilities provided to protect the experimental subject against even remote possibilities of injury, disability, or death.

8. The experiment should be conducted only by scientifically qualified persons. The highest degree of skill and care should be required through all stages of the experiment of those who conduct or engage in the experiment.

9. During the course of the experiment, the human subject should be at liberty to bring the experiment to an end, if he has reached the physical or mental state, where continuation of the experiment seemed to him to be impossible.

10. During the course of the experiment, the scientist in charge must be prepared to terminate the experiment at any stage, if he has probable cause to believe, in the exercise of the good faith, superior skill and careful judgement required of him, that a continuation of the experiment is likely to result in injury, disability, or death to the experimental subject.

Source: "Trials of War Criminals Before the Nuremberg Military Tribunals Under Control Council–Law No. 10," Vol. 2, pp. 181–182. Washington, DC: U.S. Government Printing Office, 1949.

Unfortunately, the Nuremberg Code did not prevent all ethical misconduct in human subjects research.

The Tuskegee Study of Untreated Syphilis in the Negro Male (also known as the Tuskegee Study) is an infamous study conducted by the U.S. Public Health Service that began in 1932 and ran until 1972. The study was held in Macon County, Alabama, which had the highest prevalence of syphilis in the United States at the time the study began. The majority of residents (82 percent) were Black (Baker, Brawley, and Marks 2005). Researchers believed that the complications of syphilis differed by race, and they wanted to investigate that hypothesis. This was, in the view of the researchers, a "natural lab" in which to study the effects of untreated syphilis in Black men over time. They planned to monitor the evolution of the disease through death, followed by an autopsy to determine the true extent of the disease.

When the study began, treatments for syphilis existed, but they were unreliable and quite painful (if not deadly). Because syphilis could remain dormant in the system, it often went undiagnosed and untreated until the later stages. Black men in Macon County who tested positive for syphilis were invited to take part in the study. They were told only that they had "bad blood" and that they would receive special medical treatment from the government. The study was also incentivized—participants (who were quite poor) were given free lunches, transportation, and medical treatment, $25 per year, and a $50 burial stipend (Baker et al. 2005). During World War II, these men were specifically exempted from military service so that they could remain in the study. These incentives likely helped coerce people to participate. Baker et al. (2005: 1260) quote one of the physicians involved in the study as writing, "We must remember we are dealing with a group of people who are illiterate, have no conception of time, and whose personal history is always indefinite." None of the men gave informed consent; in fact, they were misled as to what the study was about. Three hundred ninety-nine men with symptoms of tertiary syphilis were enrolled in the study. Rather than receiving the promised treatment, the men were given vitamins, tonics, and aspirin (Baker et al. 2005). Meanwhile, they were repeatedly subjected to invasive tests (such as lumbar puncture).

Following World War II, penicillin became available for the treatment and cure of syphilis, but the drug was explicitly withheld from the men enrolled in the study.

In 1964, the World Medical Association released the Declaration of Helsinki, which expanded the foundations in the Nuremberg Code to further address ethical principles for medical research on human subjects. The Declaration has since been updated and amended several times. These guidelines should have provided a halt to the Tuskegee experiment; however, it was not until 1966 that someone with the U.S. Public Health Service raised concerns about the study to the Centers for Disease Control. After years of trying to bring light to the situation, they were finally able to persuade *The New York Times* to publish an investigative story about the study. This was in 1972, forty years after the study had begun, twenty-eight years after a cure was widely available. After rounds of investigation into the ethics of the study, it was finally halted.

According to Baker et al. (2005), approximately one hundred of the men died as a direct result of their disease. It is unknown how many people contracted syphilis from the men in the study, or how many infants were born with congenital syphilis. Thirteen peer-reviewed papers were published on the study, none of which seemed to raise concern from readers about the ethics of the research. In 1997, President Clinton issued a formal apology to the few remaining survivors, and each received $20,000 from a lawsuit related to the research.

Clearly, medical research has the potential to do significant harm to participants, but what about social science research? We turn now to two famous cases, Humphrey's Tearoom Trade, published in 1970, and Zimbardo's Stanford Prison Experiment, published in 1973. Before we move to that, however, I note that although these cases are regularly used as examples of unethical human research studies, there are unfortunately many other cases (including more recent ones) that we could explore.

For his dissertation, Laud Humphreys (1975) investigated "Tearoom sex," which was a term for men performing fellatio on each other in public restrooms. He was interested in the motivations of men engaged in this practice.

At this time, men could be arrested for having sex with other men if they were caught by the police. Because of this risk, a third man would often serve as a "watch queen" to keep alert for the police and signal the men if someone was approaching. Humphries served in this role and watched hundreds of men engage in this act. He took detailed notes on their behaviors, without informing them about what he was up to.

In some cases, Humphreys was able to convince the men to participate in an interview. For those men, he disclosed what he was doing. He asked them questions about the rest of their lives, piecing together a story of men sneaking away from their wives and families to have sex with other men. In other cases, Humphries wrote down the license plate numbers of the men and used them to track down where the men lived. A year after his initial observations, he went to their homes, claimed to be a health services worker, and interviewed them about their lives. He discovered that a majority of the men were married with children and that many of them considered themselves to be heterosexual. They were simply looking for a quick, anonymous encounter.

In 1975, Humphries published a book about his findings, which became one of the best-selling books written by a sociologist. The book won the prestigious C. Wright Mills award and received positive reviews in the top sociology journals. Despite this, some scholars began to question the ethics of his study.

Although he protected the identity of his subjects, Humphries practiced deception, both in his observations as watch queen and in tracking down and interviewing the men later. Because of this deception, the men were unable to give informed consent; they had no idea that they were being studied.

One might argue that it was only through deception that Humphreys could have arrived at his findings. Indeed, there are some circumstances, particularly in psychological experiments, in which deception is allowable (Boyton, Portnoy, and Johnson 2013). In these cases, however, the participant is informed that they are taking part in a research study (and they give consent to do so), but they are not told the real purpose behind the research. Following the experiment, the participants are debriefed—told about the true purpose of the study and allowed to ask questions about their participation.

The first principle in the Nuremburg Code is that participants must be given the opportunity to give informed consent to participation in a research study. Yet most of the men in Humphreys' study had no idea they were being studied.

In addition to the matter of deception and inability to give informed consent, Humphreys also violated any sense of relational ethics, which we discuss later in this chapter.

The Stanford Prison Experiment, conducted by Philip Zimbardo and colleagues (1973), began as a study to understand whether prison brutality occurred due the personalities of the guards and the prisoners or if the way in which the prison system was set up caused those behaviors. They quickly learned the answer. It was the prison system itself, and not an individual's personality, that caused prison brutality.

Zimbardo created a makeshift prison in the basement of the psychology building at Stanford University. He then recruited volunteers to take part in the study. In his recruitment materials, he stated that he wanted to understand the psychology of prison life and that volunteers would receive $15 per day for participation. He interviewed the volunteers and rejected anyone with a previous history of criminal activity or drug abuse, anyone with any psychological or medical issues, and anyone who exhibited antisocial behaviors. Twenty-three men participated in the study. They did not know each other before the study began. Zimbardo randomly assigned each participant the role of either prisoner or guard. The study was to last for two weeks.

To make the study as realistic as possible, the "prisoners" were arrested unexpectedly at their homes. They were taken to a local police station, photographed, and fingerprinted. They were then blindfolded and transported to the "prison." When they arrived at the prison, their clothing and personal possessions were taken away. They were stripped, deloused, and issued new clothing, bedding, and a number. The clothing consisted of a long tunic with a number sewn on it (with no underwear), a nylon cap, and a chain that was locked around one ankle. From this point on, they were addressed by their numbers and required to address each other by number rather than name.

The guards wore identical uniforms and were required to wear dark sunglasses so that the prisoners could not see their eyes. They were also issued whistles and billy clubs that were borrowed from the police department. Three guards worked at a time, while the other guards were on call if needed. The guards were told to do whatever they needed to do in order to maintain order and respect from the prisoners, short of physical violence. Zimbardo watched and recorded the behaviors, and he also assumed the role of prison warden.

Only a few hours passed before the situation degraded and the guards began harassing the prisoners. The first night, the guards blew their whistles while the prisoners were sleeping, waking them to take part in "counts." Both the guards and the prisoners quickly adopted their roles and acted as if the situation were real.

The guards insulted and degraded the prisoners. They required the prisoners to do humiliating tasks, such as clean the toilets with their bare hands, or do push-ups while a guard placed his foot on their backs or forced other prisoners to sit on their backs.

The second day of the experiment, the prisoners revolted. They took off their caps, ripped the numbers from their tunics, and barricaded their cells with their beds. In response, the guards on duty called in additional guards to help. They sprayed the prisoners with a fire extinguisher to get them away from the doors. Once they had access, they stripped the prisoners of their tunics and took away their beds. They put the leaders of the revolt in solitary confinement. They also created a "special privileges" area for the "good" prisoners. These prisoners got their beds back and were given better food, which they ate in front of the "bad" prisoners.

Within thirty-six hours of the start of the experiment, one of the prisoners had an emotional breakdown. He began crying uncontrollably and exhibited signs of rage and disorganized thinking. The guards told him he was weak and that he could not quit. His emotional breakdown continued, and the researchers released him from the study. He was not the only prisoner to suffer psychological distress. By the sixth day, the interactions, harassment, depersonalization, and psychological distress had become so extreme that the researchers ended the experiment.

Zimbardo's hypothesis—that people will take on roles assigned to them—was supported. But that finding came at a significant cost to the mental health of the participants. Members of both groups—the prisoners and the guards—said they were surprised at how they acted. Despite knowing they were part of an experiment, they behaved as if it were reality, and they quickly adopted negative behaviors.

None of the researchers expected the intense reactions by the participants; however, they should have stopped the study when those reactions first emerged. Although they had agreed to participate, the prisoners did not know they would be arrested at their homes, nor were they prepared for the treatment they received following arrest. The study was designed to dehumanize them. They were both psychologically and physically tormented. As Konnikova (2015) notes, the participants knew they were being watched, yet the observers did not stop anything that was happening. This gave the guards a sense that what they were doing was correct, that they should continue their abuse of the prisoners. Zimbardo said he got caught up in his role as warden and that he found himself having a greater concern with running the prison than with the well-being of the participants.

The Belmont Report

In 1974, the United States passed the National Research Act to ensure the protection of human subjects in medical research. This law created federal oversight of research, through the National Commission for the Protection of Human Subjects of Biomedical and Behavioral Research (which investigated the Tuskegee Study). This group released the Belmont Report, which proposed new regulations for human subjects research, in 1979.[2]

The Belmont Report provides the basic ethical principles for human subjects protections in the United States. Both biomedical and behavioral research are included within the regulations. The Commission identified three basic ethical principles that should be used as an analytical framework for evaluating the ethics of research, and these are still used:

1. Respect for persons
2. Beneficence
3. Justice

Let's explore each of these principles in some detail.

Respect for Persons

The first ethical principle in the Belmont Report states that researchers must maintain a respect for persons. According to the report, respect for persons means that people should be treated as autonomous agents. People with less capacity for autonomy, such as prisoners, children, and people with low neurocognitive functioning, should receive extra protection to ensure their ethical treatment.

By autonomy, we mean that people must have the power to make their own decisions as to whether or not they want to be involved in research, without any undue influence from the researcher. Participation in research should be voluntary, and there should be no negative repercussions or retaliation for choosing not to participate. In order to make such a decision, potential participants must be provided with complete information on which to base those decisions. They need to know what the research procedures entail and what the risks and benefits are to them should they decide to participate.

Even with complete information, some people do not have the capacity to make fully informed decisions about participation in research. As researchers, we have an ethical responsibility to ensure that those people are never taken advantage of. One example of this is research on children. Children, especially young children, cannot make the decision as to whether or not to participate in research on their own. Parents or legal guardians must be fully informed about the research so that they can make an informed decision on their children's behalf. Nonetheless, children should still be allowed to express their own views on what is happening to them, and their views should be respected. Although they may not be able to fully understand the research process, procedures should be explained to children in language that they can understand. We discuss research on children in more detail later in this chapter.

Another component of respect for persons is that participation in research should be voluntary. Participants should never feel obligated or coerced into participation. For health research, we need to ensure that patients do not feel like they have to participate because they are worried they will lose health services. Students should never feel obligated to take part in faculty research. Friends and family members should not feel obligated to participate in their loved one's research projects. Researchers must be clear not only that people may decline to participate but also that they can change their minds and leave the study at any time without penalty or repercussions.

As a check and balance on this principle, we are required to ask research participants to give either written or oral informed consent before they enter a study. According to the U.S. Office of Human Research Protections (2023),

> The informed consent process involves three key features: (1) disclosing to potential research subjects information needed to make an informed decision; (2) facilitating the understanding of what has been disclosed; and (3) promoting the voluntariness of the decision about whether or not to participate in the research.

Participants must understand exactly what will happen to them if they agree to take part in the research. For example, if you plan to conduct an hour-long interview during which you ask participants specific questions about a topic, they need to know that before they agree to participate. This way they have the agency to decide if this is how they want to spend their time and energy. If you are going to ask them to take photographs or keep a diary that you will use for data, they need to know this so they can decide if that is something they want to share with you. They also need to understand the risks to participating (which we discuss later). If you plan to draw blood or take body measurements or do anything else to them, they need to have the understanding of what it is you want and have the autonomy to say no.

Researchers should explain to potential participants what the research is about, what foreseeable risks the participants assume when taking part in the research, what will be expected from them, and inform them that they may stop their participation in the study at any time. In most cases, the researcher will provide this information in a written consent form before any procedures begin, which they will allow the participant to read and will also review orally with the participant and ask the participant to sign. The participant should be given a copy of the form to keep, and the researcher will keep the signed copy for their records. This gives both parties documentation of the consent process. Signed consent forms must be kept in a secure place. If you are not using a written form, you should find another way to document that the participant understood what was going to happen and that they gave their informed consent to be part of the research (e.g., you could audio or video record the consenting process).

Both the written documentation and the oral explanation of what the research entails need to be in language and terminology that the participant can fully understand. Explanations should be clear and as jargon-free as possible. Invite participants to ask any questions they might have during the consent process.

If the consent process will be conducted in a language other than that of the researcher, the researcher needs to be certain that the information has been properly translated and that whomever is conducting the consent process understands the research and can answer any questions. In addition, researchers should be aware that among some groups, particularly some Indigenous peoples, consent is given as a group. In this case, the researcher will have to get informed consent from both the individual participants and the tribal elders or other governing body before beginning the study.

Beneficence

The second principle in the Belmont Report is beneficence. Beneficence means that researchers will ensure that the well-being of their participants is protected. We can see here how the Stanford Prison Experiment failed in this regard. We must minimize any possible harm the study might cause the participant and ensure that the benefits of the research outweigh the risks of participating in the research. The risks to the participants should not be greater than the benefits of having conducted the research. We should never cause the participants undue harm; risks should be as minimal as possible, and the participants must be informed of those risks before deciding to participate. If researchers are conducting medical or psychological tests as part of the study, the participants should be made aware of their test results as a benefit for their participation. Researchers should also have referrals for follow-up care (e.g., providing a list of health care providers or mental health resources) should the participants need it. Part of our job as human subjects researchers is to keep our participants safe.

Most social science has minimal risks to participants. We're not usually administering experimental drugs or radiating participants or performing invasive medical procedures. Nonetheless, researchers need to consider the risks their study does have and plan for how they will protect against possible risks. Although the outcomes may not seem as egregious as those of unethical medical research, social and behavioral research has the potential to negatively impact research participants. The following are some of the possible risks we might encounter:

- Psychological harm
- Violation of privacy
- Damage to reputation
- Loss of employment
- Emotional strain
- Retraumatization
- Embarrassment/humiliation
- Damage to interpersonal relationships

You may identify additional risks specific to your study.

Although social scientists often work in tandem with biomedical scientists, most of our work is not physically invasive to our participants. Unlike biomedical research, it can be difficult to quantify the risks of social science research. We seldom subject people to possible physical harm (although it's possible; for example, if confidentiality is breached, a person might be at risk of harm by another person). Risk in social science research tends to be more nebulous. Often, the risk may be no riskier than living life. When designing research projects, researchers must identify all of the possible risks to participants. If the risks are too high, the research should be reconfigured to lower the risk, or else the study should not be performed at all. For each identified risk, the researcher must determine ways to mitigate those risks (Table 2.1).

TABLE 2.1 Mitigation Strategies for Risks of Harm to Participants

Risk	Mitigation
Emotional distress	Be cognizant of signs of emotional distress. Offer breaks if needed. Offer a list of referrals to mental health care providers (including a 24/7 crisis phone number). Offer to call a friend or family member to come pick up the participant if they are distressed. Call 911 if needed.
Damage to reputation, embarrassment, loss of employment	Secure all identifiable data. Store signed consent forms separately from data. Remove identifiers from data. Assign pseudonyms to participants. Delete and purge audio/video recordings when finished with them. Maintain confidentiality. Password protect all electronic data. Keep paper data in a locked cabinet.
Loss of time	Inform the participant how long it will realistically take to engage in the study before they agree to participate. Conduct a pilot study to determine how much time will be involved.
Legal trouble	Protect confidentiality. Ensure you understand what you are legally obligated to report to the police in your jurisdiction, and inform the participant. If you are asking questions or are in situations with your participant in which illegal activities may be mentioned or witnessed, be clear with your participant (and with yourself) what you will report to the authorities and what you will keep confidential before the research begins.

We often collect sensitive information about people that they would not want others to know. For example, you may be asking questions about a medical condition, an illicit affair, or drug use. One of the important risks we must protect is confidentiality and loss of privacy.

New researchers often confuse confidentiality with anonymity. You should know the difference. Data are anonymous when the researcher has no way of identifying the participants. An example is a survey that is taken online without collecting any personal identifiers. Data are confidential when a researcher could identify the participant but keeps the identification private. An example of this is conducting a face-to-face interview with someone and then changing the identifying data in the transcript of the interview. This is done so that if anyone else reads the transcript, they would not be able to identify the participant. The data are de-identified, but the researcher still knows who the participant is. The researcher keeps that information private.

You must also think about how you will manage and store confidential information to keep it private. Think beyond just how you will store the data. What will happen to it while you are in the field? How will you keep it protected? For example, if you are going to keep field notes in a notebook, how will you store that notebook when you are not using it? If someone got ahold of your notebook, would they be able to figure out who you wrote about?

If you decide to work with a third party, such as a transcription service, ensure they also maintain the confidentiality of your data. Many transcription businesses are Health Insurance Portability and Accountability Act (HIPAA) compliant and have data security agreements; be sure that confidentiality is maintained and that your IRB is aware of everyone who handles data. The same goes if you hire a student or collaborate with a colleague.

You must also ensure secure transmission of any electronic data (such as sending audio files to someone else so they can transcribe them).

The principle of doing no harm is an ongoing process rather than a one-time event. If, as the study progresses, you determine the risks are greater than anticipated, the study should be paused, and this should be reported to the IRB. You may need to end the study or put some additional safeguards in place.

The benefits of participating in the research should be greater than the risks to the participants. In medical research, a benefit might be access to a new drug or to information about one's health. Direct benefits are often limited for the participants in social science research. Although the study may provide insight to a larger problem, or fill some gap in the literature, there is often little in the way of direct benefit for individual participants. I have found, however, that many people who have participated in my research projects say that being heard is a benefit. We take their story seriously and listen to them. Although we are certainly not therapists, sometimes the interview can feel therapeutic for the respondent.

Incentives

Some researchers choose to incentivize the research in order to recruit participants and to compensate them for their time. They might pay them a token amount of money or give them a gift card. Some researchers will enter all the participants into a drawing for a larger amount of money. You must be careful that the incentive does not become coercive, however. I've conducted a lot of research, and I've never had to use incentives to get people to talk to me. I have found that most people want to tell their story to someone who will truly listen to them. That act of *hearing* them, listening deeply, and validating their experience is enough. Although I choose not to use incentives because of the potential of coercion, other researchers disagree with me on this point, and incentives are common in some disciplines. Thus, they could be a benefit to the participant.

If you are going to offer an incentive, make sure that it is a small one so that the incentive does not coerce people to participate who might not otherwise want to do so. Be mindful of your population. Twenty dollars may be a happy bonus for some people; it might provide a meal for a family who would go hungry without it. As such, the family may feel pressure to participate, even if they don't want to, because they need the money.

If you are working with biomedical researchers, incentives can include giving the participant data from medical tests and providing them free treatment if needed. In these cases, the incentives match up to the risk of participation better than, for example, giving a gift card to a coffee shop.

Coercion

As you plan your research protocols, think about ways in which your participants might feel obligated to participate and how you can mitigate that feeling. For example, suppose a parent has given consent for their child to participate; it's still important that you consider the child's perspective. If the child is old enough, don't ask the child if they want to participate in front of the parent because they may feel pressure from the parent to take part in the study. To be sure, age and cognitive ability matter here. A seventeen-year-old will usually be able to understand what is going on more than a five-year-old will. If you're asking a friend, colleague, or lover to take part in your research, make sure they are able to comfortably say no if they wish. Don't have physicians actively recruit patients for you; patients may fear that they will be denied treatment or will be treated differently if they decline. This also applies to teachers or other professors: Students may worry that their grades will be negatively impacted by refusal to participate.

Be as straightforward as possible:

This is the study, this is what will happen to you if you are in the study, and these are the possible risks to you. Are you ok with this? There is no penalty or negative repercussions if you say no now, or if you decide during the study that you do not want to be part of it anymore.

A Special Note About Focus Groups

During a focus group, the researcher gathers individuals together to interview as a group. The researcher aims to build group synergy. Focus groups cannot be confidential because the people in the group see and hear each other during the group interaction. You can certainly ask people to keep whatever is done or said confidential, but there is no guarantee they will do so. Although you will keep your own notes and recordings private, the participants need to know that because of the group setting, confidentiality cannot be ensured.

Justice

The third ethical principle in the Belmont Report is justice. Justice involves ensuring that any one group is not burdened with the risks of participating in research. This principle also ensures that one group does not receive the benefit of most of the research at the expense of another group.

Historically, a lot of research was conducted among prisoners because they were a convenient population to access. Likewise, people living in poverty were often targeted, using incentives that would be more meaningful to them than to people with more resources. Not only is this coercive but also it puts the burden to participate in research (and to accept the associated risks) on people with less social capital.

In addition, historically most research was done on White men, which afforded them the benefits of the research. This was particularly the case for drug trials. As a result, for many drugs there is good information about how the chemicals respond in males, but much less so in women, pregnant people, and children. Many drugs are never systematically tested in pregnant people or children, and they are either not used with those populations or used off-label.

We should not target certain populations solely because they are convenient to us. We cannot target prisoners because an incarcerated population would be easy to reach—in order to conduct research with prisoners, you must have a specific reason for researching that population. This is often a problem on college campuses, where researchers continually conduct research on students because of the ease of recruitment. Researchers working with a group they are already part of should be cognizant of this as well: It is easier to reach out to friends and acquaintances instead of casting a wide net for participants, which may skew their findings.

Faculty members should pause before turning to students as research subjects. Students should never feel obligated to participate in their instructor's research. Before conducting research on students, we need to ensure that they are the right population for our study and not simply a convenient source of participants. Students also should never be coerced with promises of extra credit or have part of their grade depend on their participation in someone's research.

Academics living in college towns need to be aware of research fatigue in those communities. My own community has two public doctoral degree–granting universities, with more than 50,000 students among the two campuses. And with all these students and faculty conducting research projects, my community has been overstudied. Part of ensuring justice in research is not overburdening a community with research requests. In addition, whenever a research project goes wrong, everyone else trying to work in that community is hampered from doing so. Halseth et al. (2016: 3) write,

> These demands for participation in research breed fatigue, particularly when study results are rarely shared with the communities, and the government programs or other forms of intervention that they are intended to inspire or enhance, while possibly launched with much fanfare and hope, often fade quickly.

Most professional organizations have additional ethical guidelines, and you should become familiar with the guidelines for your discipline. These often go into more detail about ethical issues such as authorship, relationships between researcher and participant, and other issues that may arise during a research project.

Institutional Review Boards

Researchers are not on their own with regard to determining the ethics of their studies; there must also be outside review of their studies' protocols to ensure that the researchers did not overlook any ethical problems. Research protocols are the written documentation of what you plan to do in your research. In your protocols, you must detail everything that will happen to your human subject from first to last contact. These protocols are then reviewed for any ethical issues you may have overlooked, or risks you may have overlooked or underestimated, by a neutral committee.

In addition to defining the ethical conduct for researchers, the Common Rule mandates that institutions which receive federal funding for research must have IRBs to provide oversight for research involving human subjects.

Research protocols are the written documentation of what you plan to do in your research.

An IRB is a committee of people who evaluate the ethical implications of human subjects research projects. They must be a diverse group of at least five members, including someone not affiliated with your university, a scientist, and a non-scientist. Members should be well-acquainted with the law and knowledgeable about vulnerable populations. Despite guidance, ethical questions can be sticky, and the answers are not always straightforward. We use IRBs to help provide oversight, and this is partly why IRBs are composed of a committee of individuals, rather than asking one person to provide their expert feedback.

IRBs have the authority to approve or disapprove research before it begins, and they can stop research in progress. They can also ask to have a third party witness your consent process if they believe that is warranted. They are required to give you notice of these actions in writing. In addition, if there is a problem, they are required to explain the problem in writing.

But before you are given approval to conduct research on humans, you must submit an application to your institution's IRB for review. IRB applications are statements of a researcher's intended protocols and a discussion of how the researcher will address each of the ethical principles we explored above. The applications generally ask the researcher to describe how they will get informed consent (and ask for a copy of your consent form). Researchers will also be asked to identify the potential risks in taking part in the study and how they plan to mitigate those risks.

Health care researchers may find their protocols have to be reviewed by both their university IRB and a hospital or other health care entity's IRB (although it is becoming more common to share one IRB in these cases). It is important to investigate this in the planning stages of your project because this process can take a significant amount of time. Sometimes one entity will waive review with written approval of the other entity's board (e.g., a public health department might decide that university approval is enough to move forward with the research).

IRBs have three levels of review. The levels depend on the amount and type of risk to the participants. The levels also determine how many members of the IRB will read and evaluate your application. The levels are

- exempt;
- expedited; and
- full.

An exempt application is typically reviewed by the IRB chair or one other committee member and given exempt status based on their review guidelines. An expedited review is typically reviewed by one or two members of the committee. Both exempt and expedited reviews typically have a quick turnaround time. For a full review, the entire IRB committee meets face-to-face and discusses the application. Often, subject matter experts are invited to give their opinions. Sometimes the researcher will be asked to join to explain some of the details of the proposal. The full IRB usually meets on a regular basis (the IRB at my university meets once per month, with its schedule posted on the internet). Let's look at each level of review in more detail.

Some research activities meet the definition of research and use human subjects but are exempt from the regulations because they are considered to pose a minimal risk to participants. To be exempt, the risk of participation in the study is considered to be no greater than what one would experience in usual day-to-day life. Protocols for these studies must still be reviewed by the IRB, although they undergo an informal review. The IRB, not the researcher, will make the determination that the research qualifies as exempt, so when in doubt, always consult your IRB.

The following types of projects are eligible for exempt status:

- Research that involves established or common educational processes in usual settings.
- Research that involves educational tests, surveys, interviews, or public observation with at least one of the following criteria:
  - Data are recorded in such a way that no one can identify any of the participants.
  - There is no risk to the participants of criminal or civil liability, or damage to their financial standing, employment, or reputation should identifiable information be discovered.
- Benign interventions to which an informed, adult respondent agrees to.
- Secondary data analysis in which consent is not required.

In other words, projects in which the risk to participants is miniscule are eligible for exemption. The IRB should give the researcher a letter indicating that their research was exempt. Save that letter in case you need it for future reference.

Other projects are eligible for expedited review, in which one or more IRB members review the proposal without it going to the full committee. In order to qualify for expedited review, the project must present no more than minimal risk to the participants, with the largest risk being loss of confidentiality. No more than minimal risk means that the risks of participation are no more threatening than living daily life, or taking part in routine physical or psychological tests. The following are examples of projects eligible for expedited review:

- Collection of blood via finger, heel, or ear stick, or venipuncture when the amounts are small
- Noninvasive collection of biological material (such as hair or fingernail samples)
- Noninvasive medical procedures (such as weighing the participant or electrocardiogram data).
- Research involving the use of some types of pre-existing data
- Voice, video, digital, image, or other recordings
- Most surveys, interviews, focus groups, program evaluations, or quality assurance research

Most qualitative research falls into either the exempt or expedited category.

A full review is the most comprehensive and involves a meeting of the entire IRB committee. A full review is performed when the risk to the participants could result in serious physical or psychological harm or when the study population is a protected group. We discuss protected groups in more detail below, but these include prisoners, children, pregnant people (and/or their fetuses), and people who are neurocognitively unable to give consent. Examples of high-risk studies include drug and vaccine trials, experimental surgical procedures, and some psychological research. Subject-matter experts are often brought in to lend insight to the review. For example, when reviewing medical procedures, the committee might consult an outside expert on the procedures, or when reviewing research involving prisoners, a former prisoner might be invited to lend their insight.

IRBs usually have different forms to fill out for different levels of review. The IRB can ask for a higher level of review than first suggested if the IRB believes it is needed, and it can (and should) ask you for regular updates about your project.

If you are unsure what level of review you should request for your protocol review, ask the chair of your IRB for guidance. Although the purpose of IRBs is to protect research subjects, they also help protect you as the researcher from inadvertently causing harm and from accusations that you did not follow ethical procedures. In addition, many peer-reviewed journals require a statement that your protocols were approved by your institution's IRB before they will publish human subjects research.

Whereas the researcher is responsible for ethics throughout the research process, it is up to the IRB to determine whether or not a researcher's protocols meet ethical standards under the law. *It is always better to go through review than to assume that your research does not need to undergo review.* Let your IRB make that decision.

If you decide to change your research protocols after your study has been approved, you will have to amend your IRB application before moving forward with that change. The level of review of the proposed change will depend on the risk to the participants. Minor changes are typically reviewed at a low level.

Recordkeeping cannot be understated here. You should keep a copy of your approved protocols and the approval letter you receive from the IRB. You also need to keep your signed consent forms and all other confidential material in a secure location. Store the signed consent forms in a separate location from your data so that the two cannot be connected should someone get access to them.

Any recruitment materials you plan on using must also be approved by your IRB. Include all scripts, fliers, advertisements, a template for email solicitations, and other recruitment materials in your IRB application.

Qualitative researchers need to be cognizant of their impact on human subjects, and they must be ethical in their research. When human subjects are involved, the best course of action is to let the IRB review your protocols and ensure they are ethical, even if you are unsure whether or not the study meets the federal definition of research.

Special Populations

Some groups have been designated as special populations under the law and require extra protection in research. These include prisoners, pregnant people (and their fetuses), children, and people with low neurocognitive function such that they cannot reasonably give informed consent. Here, we discuss each of these populations and also the problems that arise when researchers avoid these populations.

Often, researchers will avoid studying members of vulnerable populations because of the extra precautions that are required. They may worry that such studies will not be approved by their university's IRB solely on the grounds that a protected population is involved. Unfortunately, this has led to the underrepresentation of such groups in the medical literature (particularly research involving children and pregnancy). Much drug research, for example, is not done on pregnant people or children, which means the effects of the drugs are unknown for these populations and health care providers must use their judgment regarding whether or not to prescribe the drugs. Although there are more stringent protections for vulnerable groups, we can, and should, still do research with them, when relevant.

Prisoners

Prisoners include all people being held involuntarily by the government, including people under house arrest, people in jail pretrial, and people being held at mental health facilities or drug rehabilitation centers by court order. Prisoners receive special attention under the law because of the egregious history of research on prison populations.

Before the mid-1970s, nearly all pharmaceutical research was performed on prisoners (Maron 2014). Some of this history includes twenty years' worth of dermatological research on prisoners at Holmesburg Prison in Philadelphia, which began in the 1950s (Goodman 1998). Led by Dr. Albert Klingman of the University of Pennsylvania, prisoners were paid to be test subjects for an array of products, including Retin-A, dioxin, and radioactive isotopes. They were subjected to dermatological application and biopsies. Prisoners were paid for their participation; the going rate was $10 to $300 per experiment. This is compared to the 15 to 25 cents per day pay prisoners received for working in the prison (Goodman 1998). Clearly, the compensation could be seen as coercive. In addition, the prisoners were not fully informed about what was happening to them. This was not unusual for the time period.

Because of the potential for abuse, IRBs consider whether or not the research has direct relevance to the lives of prisoners. If it does not, if prisoners are being used because of the convenience of doing so, then the research should not move forward. Although prisoners are a protected population, there are times when a research project is appropriate for that population. For example, suppose a researcher wanted to study health care delivery within a prison, or they were interested in mental illness and support services for inmates. In these cases, with proper protections, it makes sense to conduct the research among incarcerated individuals.

Because of the history of research among this group, risks to prisoners should be no more than minimal. Like any other research participants, prisoners have the right to give informed, voluntary consent. Inmates should not feel coerced to participate, and rewards such as early parole for participation are not allowed. Care should go into the offer of any incentives for participation. Incentives that appear minimal outside of the jail setting could seem coercive to inmates. In addition, prisoners may have limited access to mental health assistance, and this must be taken into account when assessing risk. How will you handle prisoners who become emotionally or psychologically distressed from your research? The IRB will want you to have a plan in place. Unlike the outside population, a researcher cannot hand an inmate a list of mental health or other support services as a means for mitigating psychological impact. Researchers should work with staff at the facility to devise means for prisoners to cope with the stress of participation in the research if needed. It is possible that the researcher will learn confidential information that the staff would like to know, such as gang membership or drug smuggling into the facility. Confidentiality needs to include discussion of what, if any, information the researcher collects will be made available to prison staff.

When the IRB reviews protocols for research on prisoners, there should be someone on the IRB with significant experience in this setting. Usually this member is a former prisoner or experienced prison advocate. In addition, many prison systems have their own IRB that the researcher may need to work through.

Researchers wishing to work with incarcerated individuals should establish a relationship with the facility before proceeding too far with their work. You will have to have the facility's buy-in to even be allowed into it, so establish that relationship early. You will need to work with the warden or superintendent to ensure prisoners' rights are protected. Even with IRB approval, however, this is a difficult population to access. Many facilities have an outright ban on research. Building those relationships early will help, but know that even with human subjects approval, you may be denied entrance.

Pregnancy

Protections for pregnant people are in place to protect the fetus. In medical research, it is difficult to untangle how medical procedures and/or medications could impact fetal development. As such, there is a lack of research on this population. If you've been pregnant, you know how difficult it is to be sick or in pain and be unable to take any medications to help with your symptoms.

It is highly unlikely that social scientists would do any research that would negatively impact the fetus; nonetheless, pregnancy does require special protections, and if you are working with pregnant people, you need to specify that in your IRB application.

You might have noticed that I use the term "pregnant people" rather than pregnant women. This is because people who are nonbinary, transgender, or who have undergone female-to-male social or medical transitions may also choose to become pregnant. To protect the dignity of the patient, you should frame the pregnancy in the manner they choose—they may identify as a pregnant man, for example. Little research has been done on pregnancy and childbearing in these situations; it is an important research topic that, like any other topic in a health care setting, should be handled with care. In this case, the terminology you use is an ethical consideration because it speaks to respect for persons.

Children

Children are a special population because they cannot legally give informed consent. We must get consent from their parent(s) or legal guardian(s). Obviously, older children will better be able to understand the nuances of what is happening to them, but they still must be offered additional protections. The age at which a person becomes legally able to consent without approval from a parent or legal guardian varies based on local law. Most often, this is at eighteen years of age; however, in some states, it is nineteen or twenty-one years. In addition, rules vary by jurisdiction as to whether emancipated minors can give their own consent to participate in research. For studies with minimal risk, only one parent needs to sign the consent form. Studies with greater risk require signatures of both parents, unless one parent has sole custody of the child or the other parent is not known or is not involved in the child's life. There are additional considerations for children who are wards of the state (including foster children); consult your IRB for assistance with this.

Parents or legal guardians have the right to give consent for children to participate in research, but children have the right to assent to participation. The research processes and procedures should be explained to children in language they can understand, and children should be able to say whether or not they want to participate. Age and maturity level need to be taken into account, of course. Young children may not be able to express assent, but if they are clearly distressed, the researcher should interpret that as dissent and stop (unless stopping would put the child's health at risk). Older children's dissent should be respected and the research not done with them, even with parental consent. A child's assent should be recorded in some manner. Older children can sign a form similar to a consent form; for younger children, you may wish to record the interaction.

Butler-Kisber (2010: 17–18) tells a story about one of her graduate students who was doing educational research with her own five-year-old child. As an attempt to get informed consent (inasmuch as a five-year-old could give it), she wrote sentences such as "I know I can stop being in Mommy's study at any time" and then asked her son to draw pictures of what they meant. This type of visual consent form is one way to help ensure participants understand their rights.

There are additional considerations for researchers who wish to conduct their studies in a public school setting. Researchers need to be aware of how laws regulating student privacy overlap with ethics regulations.

For researchers interested in studying children, working with a school seems like the perfect place to do their work. It's a convenient setting. However, school districts exist to educate children, and they will ensure children are protected from the disruption of research.

To conduct research in schools, you will need to go through multiple layers of approval. Not only do you need IRB approval but also you will likely need the approval of both the school superintendent and the principal or director of the school you wish to work in. You must also secure parental consent and child assent.

In the United States, when conducting research in an educational setting, researchers should ensure they are familiar with the Family Educational Rights and Privacy Act (FERPA) and the Protection of Pupil Rights Amendment (PPRA; also known as No Child Left Behind). FERPA grants student privacy, particularly around assessments, grades, and other school records. PPRA protects students from third-party survey research on sensitive topics.

Another thing to consider when researching with children is the difference between interviewing children and interviewing adults. It requires a different skill set that you should learn if you are going to study children. I once investigated an outbreak of coxsackievirus at an elementary school. Unfortunately, the ideal people to interview were the children (ages five to ten years). I needed to ask them what they ate for lunch the day before because we were trying to determine if this was a foodborne outbreak or not. If the outbreak was foodborne, we needed to identify which food was the cause (at that point, we did not know it was a viral infection).

Before we arrived at the school, the children had decided among themselves that hot dogs were the culprit, and they told me that. Most of the children had no idea what they had eaten the day before. Although I had the menu, they told me they had eaten all sorts of foods that had not been served. In the end, we found out that it was not foodborne at all; a sick cafeteria worker was the source.

Although interviewing young children is challenging, it does give you the opportunity to get their perspective without filtering it through an adult (Olson 2011). Olson (2011) recommends interviewing young children while they are playing. Observation may be more useful than trying to question them the way I did. Olson also notes that younger children may be more comfortable with the researcher when their parents are present. In contrast, teenagers might be more open with you when their parents are not present (especially when talking about subjects such as sexual behavior, drug use, or deviance).

Other Groups of Concern

Although people who are ill are not specifically addressed as a vulnerable population in terms of the Common Rule, because this is a book on researching health and illness, I think we should touch on this. The elderly may fall into this group as well.

People who are ill may not have the stamina for a long interview, so be cognizant of signs of fatigue. The interview may be triggering for them, for example, if you interview people about sexual assault or post-traumatic stress disorder or other traumatic experiences. Likewise, you need to make sure that you are able to handle their distress. As discussed later, you need to have resources available for them should they need follow-up care.

Some of the people you want to do research with may have cognitive impairments, for example, from illness, injury, or the medications they are taking. Ensure that they are able to give informed consent. In severe cases, you may need to seek out a legal guardian for approval for the individual to take part in research. Plan for these interviews to be longer than those with people who do not have cognitive limitations. Allow your respondents to take their time. Do not rush their answers. They may need extra time to process what it is you are asking of them.

Other people may be hard of hearing, so you'll want to ensure they can see your mouth while you talk; they may need to lip read. When interviewing someone who is deaf, you may need an interpreter.

Language

When designing your study, consider the literacy of your participants. According to the Program for the International Assessment of Adult Competencies (2013), a study of adult literacy, 52 percent of Americans read at a basic or below basic level. This means they read at a fifth-grade level or below. Many software programs are available to check the grade level of your writing. Check the grade level of your consent form. Does it match the literacy of your participants? If not, adjust the language so that it does. In order to give informed consent, your participants have to be able to understand what you are asking of them. This means you have to be able to explain it in language that is clear, precise, and understandable.

In some cases, you might wish to conduct research with people whose primary language is different from your own. It's important to consider how language impacts the research.

If you decide to work with a translator, be sure that person is well trained in your research method and in research ethics. You should consider having a third person who is bilingual double-check the translations. Even when a participant is multilingual, you should be careful to ensure understanding—theirs and yours. They may choose not to participate if they think language will be a barrier.

Language shapes what it is even possible to think. We all know about times when information was lost in translation. Once in Mexico, I saw a sign in English that said, "Do not throw your body into the pool." In other words, no diving. I have a lovely book of words in a variety of languages that do not have an English translation—the concepts the words represent aren't part of English thought. My daughter is fluent in American Sign Language (ASL). ASL is a language of concepts rather than direct translation of spoken words. Someone who speaks ASL as their primary language has a radically different thought structure than someone who speaks English.

Informed Consent

We've talked a lot about what it means to give informed consent, but let's consider some of the additional barriers to giving informed consent for people who fall outside of the protected groups.

At all times, we must treat our research participants with dignity and respect. They must have the agency to decide to what extent (if any) they want to take part in our research.

Informed consent, however, can be a complex issue. Think about how you would handle the following scenarios:

1. A participant cannot read.
2. A participant's primary language is not the same as that of the researcher.
3. A participant has a low cognitive ability.
4. A participant is unconscious.
5. A participant is a fetus.
6. A participant is in the country without permission and does not want to sign the form.
7. A participant has committed a crime and does not want to provide their real name.

You can probably think of other situations such as these in which giving informed consent is challenging. How do you ensure that in such cases participants are fully informed about the research and that they truly give consent?

The researcher must document that the participant understood and agreed to take part in the study. Usually this is accomplished with a signed consent form. In some cases, an IRB will allow for verbal consent. Such consent should still be recorded (such as with an audio recording).

When I conduct interviews, I obtain a signed consent form. I also give the participant an unsigned copy for them to keep. This way, they have information about the study and about who to contact if any problems arise. I audio record the interviews. When I turn on the recorder, I first ask them to confirm that they voluntarily chose to participate, and I reiterate that they can stop participation at any time. I then ask if they have any questions for me before we begin.

To ensure informed consent, the researcher must explain the research procedures to the participant so that they understand exactly what will happen to them and that they understand the risks and benefits of taking part in the study. They should also be told what will happen to the data—for example, that you will use de-identified quotes from their interview in publications or presentations. The explanation must be in clear, understandable terms. The participant must be given time to think about their response, without feeling pressured to make a decision about whether or not to take part in the research. They should be invited to ask any questions they might have both before and after they agree to participate.

Consent should also be an ongoing event rather than a one-time interaction. They need to know that they have the right to end their participation at any time without penalty.

The Consent Form

Your IRB probably has an example consent form that has been vetted through your university's legal department that they want you to use. The consent form should include the following:

- Explanation that this project is being conducted for the purpose of research.
- The amount of time involved in participation.
- What you intend to do to/with the participant.
- Notice if anything you intend to do or use is experimental (such as drug testing or innovative surgical techniques).
- Identification of all foreseeable risks of participation.
- Discussion of any benefits to the subject or to others that are expected outcomes of the research.
- Discussion of alternative treatments (usually this applies to biomedical research but could be appropriate for psychological research).
- A statement specifying the extent of confidentiality allowed under the law (e.g., some information, such as discussion of harm to a child, must be reported by law, trumping confidentiality protections).
- If risks are more than minimal, researchers must include information about how the participant will receive care or compensation for harm.

- Name and contact information of someone at the university other than the researcher to ask questions about the participant's rights, or to contact in case of research-related harm (often this will be someone on the IRB or in your university's research office).
- Notice that participation is voluntary and no harm will come from choosing not to participate or to stopping their participation at any time.
- A statement about how you will protect their privacy.
- How you intend to use the data.

Depending on the research, there may be additional information you want to ensure the participant has in order to give fully informed consent. Note that you cannot put language in the consent form that relinquishes their legal right to sue you if something goes wrong. Many institutions have liability insurance to cover researchers; find out the practice at your institution.

All of this information must be written in the language and at a writing level that the potential participants can easily understand.

Sample Consent Form

[NAME OF UNIVERSITY]

CONSENT TO PARTICIPATE IN RESEARCH

Title: An Exploration of Women's Use of Midwives and Home Births

Principal Investigator: Julie Smith, PhD   jsmith@university.edu (940) 000-0000

Summary and Key Information About the Study

You are being invited to take part in a research study conducted by Dr. Julie Smith, who is a professor at [name of university]. The purpose of this research is to understand women's experience giving birth at home with the assistance of a midwife.

You have been invited to take part in this research because you have had a home birth with a midwife's assistance. As a participant in this research, you will be interviewed face-to-face with Dr. Smith. She will ask you questions about your experience.

With your permission, this interview will be audio recorded, and Dr. Smith will use a code name to protect your confidentiality. The total time commitment for this study will be about one hour and 30 minutes. The greatest risks of this study include potential loss of confidentiality and emotional discomfort.

Your participation in this study is completely voluntary. You may ask questions at any time, including before or after the interview takes place. You may skip any question that you do not wish to answer. You may refuse to participate or end the interview at any time without penalty.

Description of Procedures

As a participant in this study, you will be asked to spend one and a half hours of your time in a face-to-face interview with Dr. Smith. Dr. Smith will ask you questions about your experience giving birth at home with the assistance of a midwife.

You and Dr. Smith will decide together on a private location where and when the interview will take place. The interview will be audio recorded and then written down (transcribed) so that the researcher can be accurate when studying what you have said. In order to be a participant in this study, you must be at least eighteen years of age or older and have given birth at home with the use of a midwife.

Potential Risks

Dr. Smith will ask you about your experience giving birth at home with a midwife. This will include asking about the birth and if anything went wrong with the birth. A possible risk in this study is discomfort with the questions you are asked. If you become tired or upset you may take breaks as needed. You may also stop answering questions at any time and end the interview. If you feel you need to talk to a professional about your discomfort, Dr. Smith has provided you with a list of resources.

Another risk in this study is loss of confidentiality. Confidentiality will be protected to the extent that is allowed by law. The interview will be held at a private location that you and the researcher have agreed upon. A code name, not your real name, will be used to protect your information. No one but the researcher will know your real name.

Once the audio recording has been transcribed, it will be deleted. The transcription will be labeled with the code name and will be stored in a locked cabinet in Dr. Smith's office. Only Dr. Smith will hear the audio recording or read the written interview. After the study is finished, the transcript will be destroyed. The signed consent form will be stored separately from all collected information and will be destroyed three years after the study is closed.

The results of the study may be reported in scientific magazines or journals, books, social media, or in other writing. They may be presented at scholarly conferences. Your real name or any other information that could identify you will not be included. Some of the words you say may be used in the form of a quote, but no identifying information about you will be related to the quote.

There is a potential risk of loss of confidentiality in all email, downloading, electronic meetings, and internet transactions. Dr. Smith will try to prevent any problem that could happen to you because of this research. You should let her know at once if there is a problem and she will try to help you. However, the university does not provide medical services or financial assistance for injuries that might happen because you are taking part in this research.

Participation and Benefits

Your involvement in this study is completely voluntary and you may withdraw from the study at any time. If you would like to know the results of this study we will email or mail them to you.

Questions Regarding the Study

You will be given a copy of this signed and dated consent form to keep. If you have any questions about the research study you should ask Dr. Smith; her contact information is at the top of this form. If you have questions about your rights as a participant in this research or the way this study has been conducted, you may contact the University Office of Research and Sponsored Programs at 940-000-0000 or via email at IRB@university.edu.

_____   _____

Signature of Participant   Date

If you would like to know the results of this study tell us where you want them to be sent:

Email: _____ or Address: _____

Table 2.2 is part of a transcript that includes the consenting process, as an example of how the interaction might unfold. In the transcript, PI stands for principal investigator (the researcher), and P stands for participant.

Deception

Generally, we should avoid any deception of our research participants. Deception goes against the principle of informed consent, and most IRBs will not approve deception in research.

Often, students worry that if they tell the participant too much about the research, the participant will change their answers or behavior to reflect what they think the researcher wants. And this is indeed something that can happen. It is called the Hawthorne effect (McCambridge, Witton, and Elbourne 2014).

If you are going to use deception, there must be clear reasons for doing so. Stating that people are more likely to talk to you if they don't know you're a researcher is not reason enough. You must learn to build rapport with people to get them to talk to you—not pretend

TABLE 2.2 The Consenting Process

Speaker	Text	Notes
PI	Hi! Were you able to find this place ok?	We met at the Starbucks near campus.
P	Yes, although it was difficult to park.	
PI	There are a lot of businesses in this shopping center, I had a hard time finding a spot too. Would you like something to drink?	
P	Sure.	The participant stands up to buy something, but I offer to buy it for them. After I get the drinks, I return to the table.
P	Oh, thank you.	
PI	No trouble. Now, just as a reminder, I am a professor at Texas Woman's University doing research on mothers who gave birth at home with the assistance of a midwife. Are you still interested in doing an interview?	I pull the IRB paperwork out of my bag.
P	Absolutely.	She nods vigorously.
PI	Great! Before we get started there's some housekeeping we need to do. As you know, we are doing this interview as a part of a research project. I will be asking you questions so that I can learn more about your experience with homebirth. While I will protect your privacy, I will be using some of your words in my written and oral reports about this project. Are you ok with that?	
P	Yes, that's fine. As long as my name isn't on it.	
PI	I will not use your real name. I may use a pseudonym so that it is easier to read. Because this is research, there are some risks to participating.	I hand the P the consent form.
P	Risks? What do you mean?	
PI	It's my job to keep everything you tell me confidential. I will do everything in my power to protect your privacy. If I ask you anything you don't want to answer, just say so, that's fine. If you want to take a break, or if you want to stop the interview, you can do that without any penalty. Would you like to take a moment to read through the consent form?	
P	Um, ok.	P takes a few minutes to read the form and then signs it.
PI	Do you have any questions for me before we get started?	
P	Not really.	
PI	Ok, great. If you think of any questions while we are talking, please just ask. Well, tell me then, what made you decide to give birth at home?	

you're someone you're not and trick people into telling you things. The more comfortable the participant is with you, the less likely they are to alter their behavior or responses to your questions. Most people like to talk about themselves, especially when someone else is listening closely.

There are some cases in which full knowledge of the research could bias the results, but those are rare. This sometimes arises in psychological research. If the IRB decides the deception is allowable, you must have plans in place to debrief the participant following the deception. As soon as possible, they should be informed about the deception and the reasons for it. They should also be allowed to ask questions at that time and receive complete answers.

HIPAA

Medical records are a wealth of information, but health researchers in the United States need to be aware of the boundaries that the HIPAA sets on access to medical records. An important piece of this legislation is the standards for privacy of individually identifiable health information (the HIPAA Privacy Rule) that requires health records to be kept private, although there are some exceptions to this rule.

HIPAA protects identifiable medical information, including both physical and mental health, that is collected and/or maintained by what is known as a covered entity. Covered entities include health care providers, health insurance companies, health clearinghouses, and any companies that engage in electronic medical records transmission.

For researchers, this means that we cannot access a patient's protected health information from their health care provider without the patient's express consent. This includes everything in their medical chart: patient name, date of birth, Social Security number, physical or mental health symptoms and diagnosis, treatment information, or any other information that would allow another person to identify the patient.[3]

IRB applications usually ask if the researcher intends to use protected health information and, if so, how they will address HIPAA. In order to use protected health information in research, a researcher must receive written consent from the patient to use it. In certain cases, this may be waived, but these are rare.

HIPAA does allow for review of medical records to identify potential research subjects. In this case, the researcher would ask the covered entity to review their records for particular patient characteristics. The covered entity can then tell the patient about the research project, and the patient can reach out to the researcher if they are interested in participating. This can be of direct benefit to the patient; for example, a physician might guide the patient to a clinical drug trial that could help their condition.

Researchers may use protected health information that is part of a fully de-identified data set without patient consent. De-identified data are data for which all patient identifiers have been removed and one could not realistically identify any individual patient in the data set. There are some provisions in the law for use of limited data sets, in which identifiers are removed, but there is still the possibility for identification. These require specific data use agreements between the researcher and the covered entity that provide for patient privacy.

Adverse Events

Despite all of our precautions, adverse events will sometimes crop up during a research project. You are required to report any adverse events to your IRB as soon as you learn about them, even if you think the events are minor.

Once a colleague of mine found signed consent forms laying on top of her graduate research assistant's desk. Those forms were supposed to be kept secured in a locked filing cabinet. Although the assistant said that the forms were there only a few minutes, this is an adverse event because of the possibility that someone outside of the research team saw the forms and participants' confidentiality was breached. My colleague reported the event to her IRB and then retrained the research team on confidentiality and the importance of securing paperwork.

In another instance, a different colleague received word that two days after interviewing a participant about domestic violence, that participant killed herself. Did the interview trigger the suicide? My colleague immediately reported the event to the IRB, which then stopped the study and performed an investigation into that question. The IRB reviewed the taped recordings of the interview and contacted the participant's family and local police to determine if there was any connection between the interview and the participant's death. The IRB could not find any connection, and my colleague was allowed to continue her research. Despite not finding a connection, my colleague was understandably very upset by the incident and felt responsible.

Sometimes a researcher will discover the risks to their study were greater than anticipated. An example of this might be more severe side effects than expected in a drug trial, or perhaps the interview questions proved to be too emotionally triggering to many of the participants. Our ultimate concern is always for the welfare of the people who take part in our research, and we must do all we can to protect them from harm. We need to monitor our participants' well-being during the research and report any problems to the IRB to ensure that further harm is not committed, even if that puts an end to our study.

Research Misconduct

In our discussion of research ethics, we must also discuss the issue of research misconduct. Unfortunately, this happens as well.

The Federal Research Misconduct Policy[4] defines research misconduct thusly:

Research misconduct is defined as fabrication, falsification, or plagiarism in proposing, performing, or reviewing research, or in reporting research results.

1. No rights, privileges, benefits or obligations are created or abridged by issuance of this policy alone. The creation or abridgment of rights, privileges, benefits or obligations, if any, shall occur only upon implementation of this policy by the Federal agencies.

2. Research, as used herein, includes all basic, applied, and demonstration research in all fields of science, engineering, and mathematics. This includes, but is not limited to, research in economics, education, linguistics, medicine, psychology, social sciences, statistics, and research involving human subjects or animals.

   Fabrication is making up data or results and recording or reporting them.

   Falsification is manipulating research materials, equipment, or processes, or changing or omitting data or results such that the research is not accurately represented in the research record.

3. The research record is the record of data or results that embody the facts resulting from scientific inquiry, and includes, but is not limited to, research proposals, laboratory records, both physical and electronic, progress reports, abstracts, theses, oral presentations, internal reports, and journal articles.

   Plagiarism is the appropriation of another person's ideas, processes, results, or words without giving appropriate credit. Research misconduct does not include honest error or differences of opinion.

Research misconduct involves fabrication, falsification, and/or plagiarism. Let's explore each of these in more detail.

Researchers have been known to fabricate data or results and present them as real in their publications. In a famous case that came to light in 2002 known as the Schön scandal, physicist Jan Hendrik Schön was found to have fabricated the results in seventeen peer-reviewed journal articles (Service 2002). Schön was known for his productivity: Within a four-year period, he published 90 journal articles, and he was heralded as a rising star in the field. But his fame led to close examination of his work. Fellow physicists saw inconsistencies in his articles and became suspicious of Schön's findings. A review panel discovered the data fabrication. Schön was fired from Bell Labs, where he worked, and his university revoked his PhD (Vogel 2011).

Falsification occurs when data are manipulated to show the outcome a researcher wants to achieve. In 2015, Iowa State University researcher Dong-Pyou Han was sentenced to prison and fined $7.2 million for fabrication and falsification of results from his HIV vaccine trials (Reardon 2015). Han's research had been supported with National Institutes of Health (NIH) grant funds. Han plead guilty to two felony charges of lying to obtain those grants.

Han added human HIV antibodies to rabbit blood in order to support his claims that his vaccine was causing the development of HIV antibodies (Reardon 2015). Han claimed the original contamination was accidental; however, he not only covered up the mistake but also continued to rely on that mistake to secure funding. He continued to spike rabbit blood with human antibodies for years (Phillip 2015). The falsification was discovered by researchers who tried to validate the research and found the human antibodies in the blood samples.

Plagiarism occurs when a researcher uses another person's ideas, words, processes, results, and so on without giving that person credit. University of Pittsburgh School of Nursing professor Scott J. M. Weber was found guilty of plagiarism as well as falsification and fabrication of data in 2011 (Erdley 2011). Weber's actions were discovered by a journal editor who noticed problems in his articles. The editor decided to run some of Weber's articles through an electronic plagiarism checker. The system noted that 90 percent of one of the articles and 66 percent of a second article were plagiarized from other sources. Seven articles were retracted and others in press were pulled. In addition, authorities discovered Weber had plagiarized parts of his NIH grant applications.

It is not difficult to imagine why researchers engage in research misconduct. The publish or perish adage is true in higher education, and academics often feel intense pressure to publish peer-reviewed articles or other texts. Publication is largely how we are judged as academics, and at most schools it is a major component in promotion and tenure decisions. Clearly, however, fabrication, falsification, and plagiarism are gross ethical misconduct. As we've seen, they can lead to jail time, unemployment, and the loss of one's PhD credentials.

Authorship

Many universities have policies in place about how authorship should be determined, so it is important for you to learn your own institution's policy. Generally, all listed authors need to put equal work into the project. Disciplinary conventions vary as to the order of authorship; find out what is appropriate in your field. A person should not be listed as an author as a courtesy or other honorarium if they did not do the work. Students should not feel obligated to include their professors as co-authors, unless the professors put in an equal share of the work. Writing a paper for a class and then publishing it does not automatically mean the instructor should be listed as an author; however, you should discuss it with your professor if they provided a lot of assistance with it. Disciplines vary as to whether or not one's major professor should be listed as an author on any publications generated by a student's thesis or dissertation. When working collaboratively on a research project, you should discuss authorship as soon as possible to avoid later misunderstandings.

Some Criticisms of Institutional Review Boards

Institutional Review Boards serve as auditors of research ethics. But some researchers argue that their reach goes too far. IRB guidelines were written with biomedical research in mind, and it is sometimes less clear how qualitative research fits in. Many IRB members are unfamiliar with qualitative research, especially as qualitative methodology morphs into new forms that seem more like humanities than social science (arts-based research and autoethnography are both good examples) (Lapadat 2018).

Over time, universities have witnessed what some scholars refer to as "IRB creep" (Riordan and Riordan 2009). Their scope of influence continues to grow, and committee members will sometimes focus on elements of the project that are outside of their purview (e.g., questioning the wording of an interview prompt because of personal interviewing style rather than any ethical implications). This can be frustrating to navigate as a researcher. There is often tension between trying to get started on your research and what can feel like jumping through hoops with your IRB (Halse and Honey 2007).

Universities have a bureaucratic structure that surrounds faculty and student research (Halse and Honey 2007). It is important to know the policies, procedures, and paperwork that your institution has. Halse and Honey (2007: 344) write,

> The (almost) inevitable disconnection between the technologies of ethics review and the relational ethics of "real world" research means there is always a danger that what is taken to be ethical research within institutions will be reduced to no more than a performance by researchers of a suite of textual competencies deemed necessary and desirable within the discourse's governing conditions: the ability to fill out the forms in the approved way, to deploy "ethics-speak" as required, and to couch a research project in the language of scientific objectivity that resonates with many ethics review committees.

I've also seen the bureaucratic machine of some IRBs significantly delay the start of projects over minor issues. These often have more to do with how the IRB wanted the paperwork filled out rather than anything to do with the ethics of the research.

One of my students wanted to interview people who got a certain applied college degree but who then chose not to pursue a career in that field. It was a pretty straightforward project and very low risk. In his IRB application, he wrote "adults" in the box where it asked for the age of participants. This is what I regularly do in my own IRB applications, and it was how I had advised him to fill out the form. The IRB kicked it back and insisted he put an age range instead. So he wrote 20–90, assuming that the earliest age one could complete that degree would be twenty years (even though that would be unlikely). The IRB kicked the application back to him again and asked why he was excluding people older than age ninety years. His first response to me was a sarcastic "Because they are dead? Or certainly not working in this field." We circled back to the research question—he was interested in people who got an applied degree but then chose not to work in that field. We wrote back to the IRB and explained that he was not trying to exclude nonagenarians; rather, it did not make sense that a person that age would be a member of the research population. The application was finally approved, but that process took several weeks and substantially delayed the project.

Some researchers will abandon interesting projects because they don't want to deal with the hassle of the IRB. Usually this involves research with children. They will set the age of participants at eighteen years or older for this reason, rather than work with their IRB to get the study group they want. This is unfortunate, especially because research on children is lacking.

Some qualitative researchers have challenged the notion that our work should require IRB review (Denzin and Lincoln 2018). In a joint document prepared by the American Association of University Professors (AAUP 2000), which included input from the American Anthropological Association, the American Historical Association, the American Political

Science Association, the American Sociological Association, the Oral History Association, and the Organization of American Historians, concerns were raised about IRB review and the social sciences.

First, the authors argued that the reach of the IRB has gone too far (while noting that some people believe the opposite, that it does not do enough). Second, they raised concern about the relationship between IRBs and academic freedom. Third, they noted that the application of biomedical standards of research on social sciences is not appropriate.

Most of the applications that IRBs review (approximately 75 percent) relate to clinical and biomedical research. Often, IRB members do not have a background and training in social science methods, let alone qualitative methods. Social scientists are asked to fit their research into a biomedical research model, even when such a model is not appropriate. Indeed, in most cases, the possible risks of participating in social science research are negligible compared to the risks of partaking in biomedical research. As the AAUP (2000) report states, the risks that participants typically encounter in social science research are things such as "unease, discomfort, or embarrassment," which are no different than those that people encounter in their usual daily lives. Because of this, historians lobbied to have their work, oral history in particular, exempted from having to go through IRB review. Their endeavor was successful. Some qualitative researchers argue that we should have the same leeway as historians because we are basically doing the same thing—asking people questions about their lives.

However, it is still important to consider whether or not our research could cause harm to participants. I met a woman one year at the Oral History Association's annual meeting who was collecting oral histories from soldiers returning from the war in Iraq. Although this project technically did not need to undergo review because it was classified as oral history, I believe it should have been reviewed. The context and timing of that research could have been retraumatizing to the soldiers. On the other hand, I have heard of qualitative interviews that seem so benign that even completing the IRB paperwork seems a waste of time. Either way, I think your best bet is to go through your IRB to protect both your participants and yourself.

Whereas some social scientists argue that the reach of IRBs has gone too far, some biomedical scientists argue the reach is not far enough. This is due to egregious errors that have resulted in the death of patients in the course of biomedical research.

Another concern is the potential for IRBs to impinge on academic freedom. Academic freedom is the principle that faculty members should be free to express their ideas and follow lines of research without censorship or retaliation. Although funding sources are certainly able to put parameters on the research conducted with their financial support, a significant amount of research (especially in the social sciences and humanities) is unfunded. Yet at most institutions, their unfunded work must nonetheless be reviewed by the IRB. Although they certainly don't argue for the right to harm anyone, they worry that IRB review could put a barrier on academic freedom.

I have witnessed this myself when students and faculty members censure themselves because they assume they know how the IRB will react to their ideas. For example, I have seen many researchers whose work would be appropriate for minors choose to conduct research on adults instead because of the "hassle" of getting IRB approval for work involving minors. Sometimes this type of work will be retroactive studies (e.g., "Tell me about when you were in high school"), and the data quality is thus not great. Likewise, some students will pursue projects that are exempt from IRB out of worry the review process will set them behind for graduation. Indeed, a student of mine recently spent three months—almost a full semester—going back and forth with the IRB before her application was finally approved. Her study did not put anyone at greater risk than living everyday life; she just had problems wording things the way the IRB wanted.

As noted in the AAUP (2000) document, infringement on academic freedom could extend to research that the IRB deems offensive—for example, studies that relate race and intelligence, or research on abortion. It is thus important that the IRB review the ethics of the research on human subjects—in other words, what will happen to the people who participate in the research and how do we protect them from harm—and that it does not have a say over the methodology or topic of research.

Situational and Relational Ethics

So far, we've discussed what are known as procedural ethics. Ellis (2007) writes about an ethics of care that also includes situational and relational ethics. These ethical issues typically arise after a project has begun.

Situational ethics refer to unexpected ethical dilemmas that crop up during the course of the research. *Relational ethics* involve the ethics of interpersonal interactions.

Social science research is extractive; we ask people to give us something of themselves when we conduct research (Gaudry 2011). We use their stories as data. We write about their experiences. As such, we need to honor those experiences. We must ensure we are not being exploitative. Gullion and Tilton (2020: 58) write, "Sometimes that telling does more harm than good. Sometimes it furthers colonization and exploitation. Sometimes those stories become cautionary tales. Sometimes the participants are framed as others, as deviant, as outsiders. Sometimes researchers engage in outright knowledge theft."

Although it is unlikely that qualitative research will cause physical harm to others, as we've seen, we can do psychological or emotional harm. We can also become ensconced in dilemmas that harm us and/or harm the integrity of our research.

We begin with situational ethics. As noted, these involve ethical problems that arise during the course of the project (Ellis 2007). They may be unexpected and not addressed in your IRB application. The researcher has to decide how to deal with these problems as they happen, which can be a challenge. There is not always a clear-cut answer to these problems. Suppose, for example, that during the course of a research project on drug use, you discover that a hospital laboratory worker often goes to work high. Should you tell their employer? You promised them privacy, but there's also a health and safety issue here. You are confronted with a significant situational ethical dilemma.

More often, however, you will encounter less severe situations. When I was a graduate student, I was a member of a research team that was studying the response following a tornado disaster in Oklahoma. My part of the fieldwork was in a small town that had been almost entirely destroyed. The only building still standing was the fire station, which had a large community room in which people met to plan logistics, and it served as a shared space for meals.

This happened in the summer. On my first trip into the field (my first time ever doing fieldwork), I was dressed in shorts (cutoff jeans) and a red shirt with a silver heart on it. Very casual. I walked into the building and found that it was filled with a large group of Mennonites (the Mennonite Disaster Service is a large organization that provides hands-on help after a disaster; Phillips 2015). The Mennonite women wore long, handmade cotton dresses and bonnets over their hair. Most of the men wore overalls, long-sleeved shirts, and hats. I was obviously out of place, but I wanted to talk to them about what they were doing. I needed to build rapport.

That wasn't difficult; the people were very friendly and happy to have me there, even after I explained that I was a researcher. This was around lunchtime, and they invited me to share a meal.

At first I declined. The food was for disaster victims and the responders, not for me. I didn't want to take donated food; I could go get something to eat later. But they insisted.

I stood in line, chatting with the people around me. When I got to the table where they were serving the food, someone gave me a plate with a bologna sandwich, a bag of chips, and a soda. I took the food and went and sat at a long table with a group of Mennonites.

They chatted. I eyed that sandwich. I was a strict vegetarian. Had been for more than ten years. I found myself in the middle of a situational ethics crisis I didn't know how to handle.

I ate the sandwich. I felt bad about it later, and I got sick to my stomach. But I learned more during that lunch about disaster response than I had in all my courses and reading up until that point.

While I can't say for certain, I believe that not eating the food would have killed my rapport with the group. I was an obvious outsider. I would have looked like a jerk if I had thrown away that perfectly good, donated food that was prepared by volunteers.

Stuff will happen during your research that you don't expect. People will get mad. They will cry. They will talk to you and then change their minds about what they said and want to take it all back. You'll learn things you might rather not know, personal things about people's lives, things about people not even in the room. Likewise, you will confront your own boundaries. You might get mad or cry. You might say something you later wish you hadn't.

As much as possible, try to think through how you will handle these sorts of things before you get in the field. Now that you know my sandwich story, think about how you would deal with a similar situation. Think through how you want to handle emotional outbursts (including your own). Allow yourself some grace when you don't know what to do, and do what you can to do no harm.

Burawoy (1998) writes about the power dynamics in qualitative research and ways that we must attend to them. When we conduct qualitative work, we intervene in people's lives. It is a privilege for us when people agree to take part in our research, and we must treat them with respect and be grateful for their assistance. Burawoy writes that our intervention may include aspects of domination over the participant. We certainly saw that in our discussion of coercion. People can feel compelled to participate in our research. But there are other domination effects. For example, people might feel a need to answer questions in "socially correct" ways. Conversely, there may be times when a participant holds some power over us—such as making the time to meet with us or allowing us access to certain spaces.

Another power issue Burawoy (1998) addresses is silencing. As qualitative researchers, we need to include a variety of voices and perspectives in our research and not simply talk to people we happen to like. In whatever research project we are conducting, we need to consider who should have input, who should "have the mic" as it were, whether we personally like them or not. When we do not take this action, we silence groups and individuals.

There's an added danger of silencing ideas or information that we don't agree with. In my own ethnography of natural gas extraction (Gullion 2015), I purposely silenced members of the oil and gas industry. I chose not to include their perspective. Instead, I wanted to hear from people whose voices are normally silenced in the oil and gas discourse: the impacted residents. I do, however, believe a study of fracking from the perspective of the industry would be a fruitful line of inquiry, and I noted this in my writing.

The social world is complex. Burawoy (1998) also warns us against viewing "social forces" as concrete. We should not make assumptions about people based on their social circumstances. It's too easy (and lazy) to assume that something is happening because of discrimination, the economy, or other social structures. Yes, those may be a factor, but we need to dig deeper into what is happening in any given social interaction.

This brings us to relational ethics. Relational ethics involve the ways in which we manage the interpersonal relationships that we form while conducting our research (Ellis 2007).

Qualitative researchers often spend a lot of time in the field and getting to know their participants, and sometimes collaborating with them. Even during a one-time interview, you can form a connection with someone. Sometimes participants will become our friends (or even lovers) (Wolcott 2002). Relational ethics ask us to explore how those relationships evolve and question what responsibilities we have to our participants at different levels of relationality. Smith (2005: 97) writes that "relationships are not simply about making friends . . . researchers must be self-aware of their position within the relationship and aware of their need for engagement in power-sharing processes."

Ethics don't end when the study is complete. There is also an ethics of how we present our findings. Waziyatawin (cited in Gaudry 2011: 122) invites us to

> imagine a scholar sitting before a room full of elders from the culture he has been
> studying after his first book on them has just been published. Imagine him having
> to be accountable for his methodology, his analysis, his interpretation, and his use of
> their stories. While a discussion like this between a scholar and his subjects of study
> may never occur in this formal forum, the dialog will occur somewhere.

If this scenario makes you feel uncomfortable, you may have a relational ethics problem.

Ellis (2007) has written extensively about relational ethics. While working on her doctorate, she conducted ethnographic fieldwork with a group of people she referred to as the Fisher Folk. Over time, she built relationships with the people in her study, and as they became more comfortable with her, they shared more intimate details of their lives with her. This is perfectly normal. She began to ask herself, however, what her responsibility was to those details. Should information be treated differently as we grow closer to people?

After the study ended, the participants read her published writings about them, and they were not happy with what they read. The information may have been correct, but some of it was *personal*. The ethnographic study was well done, the analysis in-depth and detailed. But they were surprised to see everything they shared revealed.

This brought Ellis to question how much of what we learn needs to be told. She writes that "relational ethics recognizes and values mutual respect, dignity, and connectedness between researcher and researched, and between researchers and the communities in which they live and work" (Ellis 2007: 4).

When we talk casually with a friend, we don't usually expect that what we say will be repeated, let alone find it in print. If it does, we might feel betrayed. Some researchers argue that we must keep a professional distance between ourselves and our participants. Others argue that it is ok to become friends with them. Human bonds are likely to form with people; we need to think about how to manage those bonds. Smith (2005) and Bhattacharya (2007) both argue that informed consent is not a one-time action but, rather, should be fluid, revisited, revised as needed over the course of a research project. When working with people over time, remind them what it is you are doing so they aren't caught off guard later.

I once had lunch with a key informant in one of my own research projects. When she arrived at the restaurant, she gave me a hug. Then she backed away and said, "Can I do that? Can I hug you if I am one of your research specimens?" We laughed about her choice of words, but then we did talk about the fact that I was doing research, and she was part of that research.

Bhattacharya's (2007) writings on relational ethics add another dimension to the issue—that is, what to do when participants put what might seem like too much trust in your work. During a research study, Bhattacharya invited a participant to read what she had written about her to make sure that the participant was comfortable with what Bhattacharya had written. This practice is called member checking, and it is common in qualitative research. Instead of reading it, the participant told Bhattacharya that she trusted her. As an ethical researcher, this made Bhattacharya uncomfortable and not entirely sure how to handle the situation.

"The bad news," Ellis (2007: 5) writes,

> is that there are no definitive rules or universal principles that can tell you precisely what to do in every situation or relationship you may encounter, other than the vague and generic "do no harm." The good news is that we are accumulating more and more stories of research experiences that can help us think through our options.

Ethical problems are seldom straightforward. "First, do no harm" should be our mantra. Research ethics are a social justice issue. We must always uphold high ethical standards in our research. And when in doubt, we should consult with our IRB.

Notes

1. https://www.ushmm.org/information/exhibitions/online-exhibitions/special-focus/doctors-trial/nuremberg-code.
2. hhs.gov/ohrp/regulations-and-policy/belmont-report/read-the-belmont-report/index.html.
3. https://searchhealthit.techtarget.com/definition/HIPAA.
4. https://ori.hhs.gov/federal-research-misconduct-policy.

References

American Association of University Professors. 2000. "Institutional Review Boards and Social Science Research." Accessed November 20, 2019. https://www.aaup.org/report/institutional-review-boards-and-social-science-research.

Baker, Shamim M., Otis W. Brawley, and Leonard S. Marks. 2005. "Effects of Untreated Syphilis in the Negro Male, 1932 to 1972: A Closure Comes to the Tuskegee Study, 2004." *Urology* 65, no. 6: 1259–1262.

Bhattacharya, Kakali. 2007. "Consenting to the Consent Form: What Are the Fixed and Fluid Understandings Between the Researcher and the Researched?" *Qualitative Inquiry* 13, no. 8: 1095–1115.

Boyton, Marcella H., David B. Portnoy, and Blair T. Johnson. 2013. "Exploring the Ethics and Psychological Impact of Deception in Psychological Research." *IRB* 35, no. 2: 7–13.

Burawoy, Michael. 1998. "The Extended Case Method." *Sociological Theory* 16, no. 1: 4–33.

Butler-Kisber, Lynn. 2010. *Qualitative Inquiry: Thematic, Narrative and Arts-Informed Perspectives*. Los Angeles: SAGE.

Denzin, Norman K., and Yvonna S. Lincoln. 2018. "Introduction: The Discipline and Practice of Qualitative Research." In *The SAGE Handbook of Qualitative Research*, 5th ed., edited by Norman K. Denzin and Yvonna S. Lincoln, 1–26. Los Angeles: SAGE.

Ellis, Carolyn. 2007. "Telling Secrets, Revealing Lives: Relational Ethics in Research with Intimate Others." *Qualitative Inquiry* 13, no. 1: 3–29.

Erdley, Deb. 2011. "Ex-Pitt Professor Given Sanctions for Plagiarism." TribLIVE. Accessed September 11, 2019. https://archive.triblive.com/news/ex-pitt-professor-given-sanctions-for-plagiarism.

Gaudry, Adam J. 2011. "Insurgent Research." *Wicazo Sa Review* 26, no. 1: 113–136.

Goodman, Howard. 1998. "Studying Prison Experiment Research: For 20 Years, a Dermatologist Used the Inmates of a Philadelphia Prison as the Willing Subjects of Tests on Shampoo, Foot Powder, Deodorant, and Later, Mind-Altering Drugs and Dioxin." *The Baltimore Sun*. Accessed September 11, 2020. https://www.baltimoresun.com/news/bs-xpm-1998-07-21-1998202099-story.html.

Gullion, Jessica Smartt. 2015. *Fracking the Neighborhood: Reluctant Activists and Natural Gas Drilling*. Cambridge, MA: MIT Press.

Gullion, Jessica Smartt, and Abigail Tilton. 2020. *Researching with: A Decolonizing Approach to Community-Based Action Research*. Rotterdam, the Netherlands: Brill/Sense.

Halse, Christine, and Anne Honey. 2007. "Rethinking Ethics Review as Institutional Discourse." *Qualitative Inquiry* 13, no. 3: 336–352.

Halseth, Greg, Sean Markey, Laura Ryser, and Don Manson. 2016. *Doing Community-Based Research: Perspectives from the Field*. Montreal, Quebec, Canada: McGill-Queen's University Press.

Humphreys, Laud. 1975. *Tearoom Trade: Impersonal Sex in Public Places*. New York: Routledge.

Konnikova, Maria. 2015. "The Real Lesson of the Stanford Prison Experiment." *The New Yorker*. Accessed June 6, 2020. https://www.newyorker.com/science/maria-konnikova/the-real-lesson-of-the-stanford-prison-experiment.

Lapadat, Judith C. 2018. "Collaborative Autoethnography: An Ethical Approach to Inquiry That Makes a Difference." In *Qualitative Inquiry in the Public Sphere*, edited by Norman K. Denzin and Michael D. Giardina, 156–170. New York: Routledge.

Maron, Dina Fine. 2014. "Should Prisoners Be Used in Medical Experiments?" *Scientific American*. Accessed September 11, 2020. https://www.scientificamerican.com/article/should-prisoners-be-used-in-medical-experiments.

McCambridge, Jim, John Witton, and Diana R. Elbourne. 2014. "Systematic Review of the Hawthorne Effect: New Concepts Are Needed to Study Research Participation Effects." *Journal of Clinical Epidemiology* 67, no. 3: 267–277.

National Archives and Records Administration. 2018. "Common Rule." Accessed September 6, 2020. https://www.ecfr.gov/cgi-bin/retrieveECFR?gp=&SID=83cd09e1c0f5c6937cd9d7513160fc3f&pitd=20180719&n=pt45.1.46&r=PART&ty=HTM.

Olson, Karin. 2011. *Essentials of Qualitative Interviewing*. Walnut Creek, CA: Left Coast Press.

Phillip, Abby. 2015. "Researcher Who Spiked Rabbit Blood to Fake HIV Vaccine Results Slapped with Rare Prison Sentence." *The Washington Post*. Accessed September 11, 2019. https://www.washingtonpost.com/news/to-your-health/wp/2015/07/01/researcher-who-spiked-rabbit-blood-to-fake-hiv-vaccine-results-slapped-with-rare-prison-sentence.

Phillips, Brenda. 2015. *Mennonite Disaster Service: Building a Therapeutic Community After the Gulf Coast Storms*. New York: Lexington Books.

Program for the International Assessment of Adult Competencies. 2013. "Literacy, Numeracy, and Problem Solving in Technology-Rich Environments Among U.S. Adults: Results from the Program for the International Assessment of Adult Competencies 2012." Accessed September 12, 2020. https://nces.ed.gov/pubsearch/pubsinfo.asp?pubid=2014008.

Reardon, Sara. 2015. "U.S. Vaccine Researcher Sentenced to Prison for Fraud." *Nature* 523: 138–139. https://www.nature.com/news/us-vaccine-researcher-sentenced-to-prison-for-fraud-1.17660?WT.mc_id=TWT_NatureNews

Riordan, Diane A., and Michael P. Riordan. 2009. "IRB Creep: Federal Regulations Protecting Human Research Subjects and Increasing Instructors' Responsibilities." *Issues in Accounting Education* 24, no. 1: 31–43.

Service, Robert. F. 2002. "Bell Labs Fires Star Physicist Found Guilty of Forging Data." *Science* 298, no. 5591: 30–31.

Smith, Linda Tuhiwai. 2005. "On Tricky Ground: Researching the Native in the Age of Uncertainty." In *The SAGE Handbook of Qualitative Research*, 4th ed., edited by Norman K. Denzin and Yvonna S. Lincoln, 85–107. Thousand Oaks, CA: SAGE.

United States Holocaust Memorial Museum. 2006. "Nazi Medical Experiments." Accessed September 6, 2020. https://encyclopedia.ushmm.org/content/en/article/nazi-medical-experiments.

U.S. Office of Human Research Protections. 2023. "Informed Consent FAQs." Accessed September 15, 2023. https://www.hhs.gov/ohrp/regulations-and-policy/guidance/faq/informed-consent/index.html#:~:text=The%20informed%20consent%20process%20involves,to%20participate%20in%20the%20research.

Vogel, Gretchen. 2011. "Jan Hendrik Schön Loses His Ph.D." *Science*. Accessed September 11, 2019. https://www.sciencemag.org/news/2011/09/jan-hendrik-sch-n-loses-his-phd.

Wolcott, Harry F. 2002. *Sneaky Kid and Its Aftermath: Ethics and Intimacy in Fieldwork*. Walnut Creek, CA: AltaMira.

Zimbardo, Philip G. 1973. "On the Ethics of Intervention in Human Psychological Research: With Special Reference to the Stanford Prison Experiment." *Cognition* 2, no. 2: 243–256.

FURTHER READING

Iphofen, Ron, and Martin Tolich, eds. 2018. *The SAGE Handbook of Qualitative Research Ethics*. Thousand Oaks, CA: SAGE.

Wolcott, Harry F. 2002. *Sneaky Kid and Its Aftermath: Ethics and Intimacy in Fieldwork*. Walnut Creek, CA: AltaMira.

Discussion Questions

1. Why should we be concerned with ethics in research?
2. How do IRBs both help and hinder research?

Active Learning

1. Find your university's IRB application online. Practice filling it out for a project you would like to conduct. Identify all of the potential risks to participants and note how you would mitigate them.
2. Invite someone from your university's IRB to come to class and explain what the IRB looks for in an application.
3. Take your university's IRB training, if available.

Mindfulness Exercises

1. How might you cope with a participant's distress? What could you do to be more prepared for strong emotions from them?
2. What are ways that you can cope with your own emotions during an interview and about your project as a whole?

Study Design

In order to have a quality study, researchers must create a quality study design. In this chapter, we explore how to do that. We begin with a discussion of the importance of research questions and how those questions guide our research. We then think about the literature that is related to our research questions. Next, we get into the details of study design, including choosing a data collection technique, determining the unit of analysis, sample size, the issue of time and time frames, and place. Finally, we explore different ways to collect a sample of people to participate in the study and how to fund your research.

All research begins with a question. There is something that you want to know (otherwise you wouldn't be doing research), and you need a way to find out the answer. This question is called your research question, and it is the backbone of every decision you make during the course of your research project.

Once you've chosen a research question, there is a series of issues you will want to address in order to find the answer to your question:

1. What research has already been done on this topic?
2. How will you conceptualize the terms in your research question to make them measurable?
3. What data (information) do you need in order to answer the research question?
4. Who or what has the information that you need?
5. How will you get that information?
6. How will you analyze the information once you have it?
7. How will you know that you have answered your research question?

The answers to these questions help you design a research project. In this chapter, we work through this process.

Qualitative Research in Health and Illness. Jessica Smartt Gullion, Oxford University Press. © Oxford University Press 2024.
DOI: 10.1093/oso/9780190915988.003.0004

Writing a Research Question

Let's begin with how to write a research question and conceptualize the terms within the question. Suppose you are interested in how health care workers dealt with the stress of working during the COVID-19 pandemic. We begin with that question:

How did health care workers cope with the stress of working during the COVID-19 pandemic?

Now let's parse out that question. There are some key terms that we need to conceptualize (define) and operationalize (find a way to measure). That is, we look at the terms within the question and we decide how to define them and place parameters on them for measurement.

Health care workers—Specifically, which health care workers are you interested in? Physicians? Nurses? Aromatherapists? Veterinarians?

Coping with—What do you mean by this term? How do you define coping? How are they coping at work? At home? With their children and families? How do you know if someone is not coping well?

Stress—Emotional stress? Physical stress? Work-related stress? Work–life balance? What specifically do you want to know? How will you measure how much stress they are under?

Of working during—Are you interested in health care workers who work in hospitals? Or a clinic? School nurses? Pharmacists? Anesthesiologists? Do you want to talk to health care workers who took care of COVID patients? Or who didn't work directly with COVID patients?

The COVID-19 pandemic—Delineate the time period and place you are considering.

Specificity will help you focus your research and make decisions about how to structure your research design. You will also want to consider the theoretical framework (or lens) that you will use to explore your question.

Let's consider another example. In this one, suppose you are interested in the experience of women who had traumatic birth experiences. What is it about that experience you want to know? It would be important for you to define what you mean by "traumatic birth experience." One way to conceptualize this phrase is to look at the literature that has already been published on this topic. More than likely, there is an established definition for this term that other researchers use.

From the very start of your project, keep field notes and analytic memos. How you do this is up to you, but it is a crucial component of the research process. Keep notes on what decisions you make, when, and why. If you don't, you may forget why you made certain decisions, the details of what happened, and ideas that came to you at odd moments (like in the shower or while driving). We will talk much more about field notes and memos later, but for now here is a simple explanation.

Field notes are observations that you make about your project. For example, let's use the above research question about COVID-19. Suppose you decided to focus on school nurses and how they handle children who come into their clinic sick with COVID-19 symptoms, or parents who call in to the office from home and say their children have been confirmed to have COVID-19. At this point in the research, you would want to write down those parameters and how you arrived at them. You could also begin jotting down potential interview questions or ideas about how to recruit school nurses.

Analytic memos are where you work with your theory and generate theoretical insights. As your project unfolds, you will begin to have ideas about what is happening here. Maybe you discover that school nurses are being left out of the larger school district COVID-19 planning. Why is that? Jot down your thoughts here. Note ideas of what theoretical lens you will be using to study this phenomenon, and ideas about how that theory might inform your data collection. Write about theory and how it is influencing what you see.

The idea behind both field notes and analytic memos is that you keep extensive records about the process of research so you don't forget the analytic moves you've made. These are also part of your data, and they will be invaluable when you write up the results of your research.

In some projects, the research question may be broad at first and then narrow over time. For example, I conducted an ethnography about what I called reluctant activists (Gullion 2015). These were people living in North Texas on the Barnett Shale, an area rich in natural gas deposits, who became activists after learning that fracking was harming their health and well-being. When I started the project, my research question was simply, What is happening here? I delineated a geographic area in which I would conduct my work. As I spent more time in the field, I began to ask more specific questions, such as, How does one become an environmental activist? or, How does someone learn how to effectively protest?

These questions guided me to my research method. Take, for example, the question of how someone becomes an environmental activist. Because the larger focus of the project was on natural gas drilling in North Texas, the research question would then be: How did the environmental activists working on gas drilling in North Texas become activists? The best way to answer this question would be to find some environmental activists doing this work and ask them.

Reviewing the Literature

Reviewing the literature—reading what other researchers have already written on and around your research question—can help you refine your research question, teach you what is already known about this question, and help you identify what still needs to be studied about this question. Sir Isaac Newton is credited with the oft-repeated quote, "If I have seen further than others, it is by standing on the shoulders of giants." The giants are the writers who came before you. Know what they know; stand on their shoulders.

Every semester, students ask me how many sources they need in their literature reviews. My answer is always the same: All of them.

I understand this sounds daunting. After all, a quick search of many topics reveals hundreds, if not thousands, of results.

To be a scholar is to be part of an academic conversation about a particular topic. By "conversation," I don't mean a face-to-face talk with your professors. I mean a conversation through professional presentations at conferences and publications in peer-reviewed outlets (journals and books). This is one reason why reading broadly is so important. One must know what the conversation is before one can join it. One must also know the conversation if you want to make an original contribution to the discussion.

For graduate students, the thesis or dissertation is usually their entrance into that scholarly conversation. The extended formats of these projects allow students to dig into the literature, to give themselves time to understand the conversation, and to make an original contribution to it.

This is also why students and faculty are encouraged to have a clear research agenda that lasts several years of their careers, if not encompassing the totality of it. It allows them not only to stay current in their particular intellectual conversation but also to eventually become recognized as a leader of that conversation.

Find a mentor to help you begin sketching out your research agenda. For graduate students, this mentor is usually their major advisor, or chair of their thesis/dissertation. This person should be able to help you navigate the literature. If you don't have a mentor, now is a good time to find one. I guide my own students to articles that I expect to see cited in their work, and when I come across items that could be of use to their projects, I forward them to my students. I can do this because I am part of the conversation they wish to join. Ask your mentor to do the same, if they are not already doing so. This is also why you need to find a mentor who works in the same area you do, as opposed to just finding someone you like to mentor you. They should help you become part of the scholarly conversation about your topic of interest.

A literature review can help develop and refine your research question, and it can also stop you from spending a lot of time on a question others have already answered. A thorough review of the literature shows where you can put your own spin on the topic or where there are gaps in what is known about the subject that you can work to resolve.

When beginning your literature review, I suggest you make an appointment with a reference librarian at your university library. This is even more important if you do some preliminary searches and think that there isn't any literature relevant to your topic. A reference librarian is a skilled professional who knows how to access databases in ways we may never consider. Make an appointment with one, explain your project to them, and work with them to identify the relevant literature for your project.

I once worked on a project on scleroderma. I had a difficult time finding any information. Every database has a unique way of cataloging information, and if you don't understand how the database works, you may end up using the wrong keywords, which was happening to me. I complained that I could not find much previous research, which led me to think this might be groundbreaking work. It wasn't. My reference librarian came back with more than 9,000 citations related to the disease. Granted, most were not relevant to my particular study, but it gave me a jumping off place relative to the small handful of citations that I had identified on my own.

On the other hand, it can be easy to feel overwhelmed by the literature. I went to Google Scholar and searched for "cancer patients." I got back 4.9 million results. Does this mean everything has already been written about cancer patients, and people wanting to work on this topic should abandon it? Certainly not. But if this is something you are interested in, you need to find an "in" to the conversation and determine how your unique perspective can contribute to that conversation. Usually you can do this by focusing on one aspect of the subject.

Even in a playing field of 4.9 million citations, you can contribute something. I have found that if I give all the students in my research methods course a stack of the exact same articles and ask them to write a literature review and a research question using them, everyone will turn in something different. This is because the researcher brings something of themself to every project, and that something is worthwhile. We will talk more about this later in the book when we discuss standpoint, reflexivity, and diffraction. Suffice to say at this point, a piece of you is in all the research you do.

There's a meme that floats around academic corners of the internet that says something along the lines of, "I culled through fifty abstracts to find fifteen articles that I read to write one sentence." Expect that you will read much more than you think you may need to. Do not think you can use the first handful of citations you discover and be done—many of those may not even be relevant to your work.

A literature review sets the context for your study, but it should be more than a litany of previous work of your topic. You don't want to end up with paragraphs that say, study X said this, study Y said that, study Z said this. Your literature review should be a critical analysis of previous work. Demonstrate what came before, but more important, synthesize that content. One way to do this is to organize your literature review by themes or subtopics. This way, your reader can follow the logic of your argument and understand how and why you conducted your research the way you did, even if they are less familiar with the subject.

One practical consideration is how you will manage the material aspects of research, such as the articles that you find. Some scholars use qualitative data management software to store journal articles. Similarly to coding data, they create codes for their articles. They might create codes about a particular method or theory, or demographics about the subject. It's up to you to decide what you need to find again in your stash of articles. You can then have the software create a document with only the highlighted citations. Many e-book readers allow you to do something similar—everything that you highlight in your e-reader can also be downloaded into one document.

Some people prefer to read paper copies instead of working online. They may use highlighters or colored markers or write on the documents. This is what I tend to do, and the articles end up in big stacks in my office. It is not the most efficient means for working, but it is what works for me. I also keep a notebook for every literature review I work on. I write the citation for the article I'm reading, and then I write my notes about the article and direct quotes with page numbers. It is not electronic, but at least everything is contained in one place. You can use the same procedure electronically.

Other people keep an extended bibliography in a word processing document or spreadsheet. They add to it over time and use the computer's search function to find specific items. One scholar I know keeps what she calls "dictionaries." These are files about specific writers. For example, she has a dictionary of Foucault and another of Barad. When she reads their work or something about their work, she adds notes and quotations to her dictionary about them. You could do something similar for any topic. These could also be useful references when you are teaching those topics.

As with any search for information, you should remain cognizant of where the information you use is coming from. Valid information can come from all sorts of places, but you should still be mindful of the source. Although open access journals allow more people to access academic knowledge, it can be difficult to distinguish between legitimate and predatory journals. This is another reason it is helpful to consult with a reference librarian; they should be able to tell you the quality of the journals you're reading.

You should also be mindful of the date of the publication. Times change, and what happened long ago may not be relevant now. Some scholars use older studies as a method for coming up with research ideas—they replicate older studies to see if and how things have changed over time. Philosophical and theoretical texts may be much older; however, be sure to read how others are working with those ideas in the present and the ways in which the original ideas have been shaped and interpreted over time. You want to demonstrate that you are knowledgeable about the current research in your field and not have your work rejected because you missed an important piece of scholarship.

When you begin this process, you will spend a lot of time trying to sort through information that may be new to you. When you encounter ideas that you don't understand, search for more information on them. Also make use of the references in the text you are reading. Go back and read the articles that an author cites to understand the foundation of that author's argument. Other writers' reference lists are a great way to find articles that are also relevant to your topic.

There is some debate among qualitative scholars as to when one should conduct a literature review. Most people do it before embarking on their research because it helps to have the background to shape what they are going to focus on. Some scholars, however—especially some ethnographers—suggest that you wait until after you return from the field so that you are not unduly influenced by what came before. They argue that the researcher should look at the scenes with "fresh" or "beginner's" eyes. A drawback to this approach is the possibility of wasting one's time reformulating ideas that are already well-established or missing important insights other scholars have written about.

There are some standardized ways to conduct meta-reviews on literature, such as the PRISMA method or the Cochrane method. They are beyond the scope of this book, but I've included some references at the end of the chapter for you in case you would like to learn more about them. Systematic meta-reviews are both useful and publishable. Many journals will accept this type of review.

Choosing a Method

Once you've decided what you plan to study, you must figure out how you are going to study it. What are the best techniques for getting the empirical materials you need to answer your research question? These techniques are your research methods.

TABLE 3.1 Common Qualitative Methods

In-depth interviews	Asking individual participants questions or talking to them about the research question.
Focus groups	Like in-depth interviews, only with a small group of people. The group works synergistically to respond to questions/prompts from the facilitator.
Observation	Watching a group or activity as an outsider.
Participation	Taking part in the phenomena of interest.
Content analysis	The study of human-created artifacts (e.g., newspapers, music, blogs).
Visual	The use of photography or video.

Typically, researchers create some sort of tool for data measurement (Table 3.1). For example, they might write a list of questions to ask a participant in an in-depth interview. Or they might create a systematic manner to collect images. Research methods are tools in your researcher toolbox. Choose the method that will best answer your question. If a method that works well for you doesn't exist, make up your own method. Use more than one method if that helps. The point is that we want to have a systematic way of collecting empirical materials (or data) that will help us answer our research question.

The measurement tool, in whatever form, shapes what the researcher is able to learn about their subject. Your measurement tool might be a list of questions or a standardized codebook for analyzing images, for example. And don't forget about your theoretical lens—whatever tool a researcher creates should be theory-informed.

The instrument we decide to use to provide us with information about our research question is not passive but, rather, is an active component of the research itself (Barad 2007). The instrument produces the data that will help us answer our research question. Data are not "out there" for us to "find" (St. Pierre 2013). Rather, we create data when we define something as such. "Every measurement involves a particular choice of apparatus," Barad (2007: 115) writes, "providing the conditions necessary to give meaning to a particular set of variables, at the exclusion of other essential variables, thereby placing a particular embodied cut delineating the object from the agencies of observation."

The instrument you choose is important to your project. The instrument helps you make meaning and understand the phenomena you are studying. And different instruments can give you different kinds of information. As Gullion (2018) notes,

> We can use vision as a simplified example of the influence the measurement instrument has on the outcomes and meanings of measurement. The human eyeball contains three different types of cones that allow us to see colors at different wavelengths. For simplicity sake, these typically are said to correspond to the red, blue, and green spectrums. Other animals have different numbers and types of cones. As such, their perception of color would be very different from ours—their measurement instrument differs. Spiders, bees, and other insects have cones that allow vision on the ultraviolet spectrum, not visible to humans. Reptiles have cones that allow vision in the infrared spectrum. While humans can perceive about 10 million colors, some species of butterflies and birds have five different types of

cones, allowing for the perception of closer to 10 billion colors. In this case, the measurement instrument (the eyeball) determines how reality is visualized and the meanings placed on the realities they reveal.

Unit of Analysis

The unit of analysis is the primary "thing" that you collect information about/from. Most often, your unit of analysis will be individuals, groups, organizations, or artifacts. The unit of observation is the subunit within the unit of analysis.

In a study on cancer, your unit of analysis could be individuals, and your subunit could be oncologists. Or people getting cancer treatments. Or it could be cultural artifacts. You could study cancer blogs. Or comedy sketches about cancer. Think through your unit of analysis and make sure it aligns with your research question. Identify who or what is in your study population as well as who or what should be excluded. Also note that your unit of analysis doesn't have to be people. It can be phenomena, concepts, or other collections.

As another example, suppose you are working on a project on handwashing among health care workers in hospitals. You could interview hospital infection control professionals to get their impressions of how well and how often hospital staff engage in handwashing. You could conduct observations, perhaps by shadowing different health care workers and watching how often they clean their hands (although they would probably be more likely to do it given you are watching them). Your unit of analysis could be infection control professionals, or it could be health care workers with direct patient care. Whomever you decide to work with, they should be the best people to answer your research question. Returning to our example of handwashing in hospitals, one population you could interview is patients; however, patients might not see the health care workers wash their hands if it's done outside of their view (e.g., if there is an alcohol-based hand sanitizer mounted on the wall outside of the exam room). Identify the population of people or things that are best positioned to help you answer your research question.

Sample Size

In statistical research, the N-size, or number of cases in the study, is of utmost importance. It influences the validity of the statistical tests that are used. Assumptions of particular statistical tests rest on the number of cases one has. There are statistical tests called power analyses that help researchers determine how many cases they need for their particular study.

Qualitative researchers do not have this same requirement. Case study research, for example, can have as few as one participant and still be valid.

The answer to the question of how many people you should interview is as simple as it is annoying: It depends. Many qualitative researchers argue that you should continue to interview people (or collect new data) until you reach data saturation—that is, until you are no longer getting any new information with additional cases. Typically, I advise my students that once they reach data saturation, they should identify one or two more people to interview (or cases to look at) who are different from the other participants and see if they get any new information. If they don't, they can stop interviewing.

There is also the difference of depth in qualitative research. An interview that lasts thirty minutes is likely to be much less informative than one that lasts three hours. Multiple interviews with the same individual over time will provide more depth than interviewing them once. Rather than worry about how many people you interview, it might be more helpful for you to examine total minutes of interview time across your study.

Unfortunately, there is no good way to predict how much data you will need in advance. Despite this, many Institutional Review Boards ask for the expected number of cases you will have in your study. As you become more experienced, you will get a better sense of how many cases you might need for a particular project, but it is still difficult to know for certain.

Time

Another variable we take into consideration in research is the time frame that you want to study. Many researchers interview people once. This gives the participant a chance to tell their story, but it does not allow the researcher to watch that story evolve over time. Other methods, such as ethnography or community-based action research, give the researcher a chance to watch processes unfold and to see how things change over time.

Bound time in your study, and be clear about what time frame you will be exploring. Time itself is arbitrary: The study begins when you enter the field and ends when you leave. You always enter and exit somewhere in the middle of people's lives. Because there is usually no discrete beginning or ending to any phenomena, you have to set them yourself.

Another consideration when thinking about how time factors into research is how memories are interpreted and stories evolve as time passes. Details tend to be forgotten, and people tend to ascribe different meanings to events after they happen. The more time passes, the more the individual has reinterpreted and inscribed different meanings onto the event. This is a significant problem in epidemiological studies, when a researcher needs mundane information to determine the source of an outbreak.

As an example, think about asking people about the experience of giving birth. The response that you get in the first week after the birth will be different from that given after one year. Details will have been forgotten. Some aspects may be blurry. Now imagine asking the same questions after ten or twenty years. You will probably hear a different story. If your questions are about an event or experience, consider the influence of the passage of time and how much time passage is acceptable to you. As another example, if a researcher was interested in nursing care in the 1970s, they could conduct an oral history project to get broad information. The participants likely would not have specific details to share, simply because those details were forgotten. This does not mean it would be a bad study. The researcher will still learn about what happened—they just need to be cognizant of how time and memory work against each other.

Place

Just as we put temporal boundaries on our projects, we also need to put geographic boundaries on them (this can include virtual boundaries as well). Your research question should guide this. In my fracking ethnography, I decided the geographic boundary would be the Barnett Shale in North Texas and Austin, Texas (because that's where the governmental regulatory agencies are). I did not interview people living or protesting at other natural gas drilling sites; they were outside of the boundaries of my study. This does not mean that people outside of the boundaries had nothing valuable to offer. I delineated the geographic boundaries because I believed that people in that area may have had common experiences (they fall under the same laws, the same regulatory agencies, and share culture).

Do you want to study something in your local community? Nationwide? In a different country from where you live? For research on the internet, do you only want to look at posts on a single discussion board? Or multiple boards about the same topic? Maybe you want to look at usage of one particular app. Be clear about the parameters and boundaries of your study, and don't go outside of them unless there's a compelling reason to do so.

Qualitative projects can get huge very quickly. The amount of empirical materials you will collect can be staggering. Putting boundaries on your research will help protect you from becoming overwhelmed and will help you to keep the project manageable. When you come across something of interest that is outside of your boundaries, make note of it for a possible future project and move on.

People

Once you have a good grasp of how you are going to answer your research question, you will engage the people who can help you answer it. Whom do you need to talk to in order to get the information you need to answer your research question? How will you get access to those people? How will you recruit them to take part in your research?

In statistical studies, a researcher selects a random sample of people from a population of people they wish to generalize to. That is the foundational assumption of statistical tests; most statistical tests are not valid if a random sample was not used. In most instances, qualitative research does not rely on random sampling because we are not trying to generalize to any particular population (of course, you can do so if you choose, but it is not common practice). Instead, our sampling tends to be purposive. We invite people to participate in our research who have particular characteristics that we are interested in.

For example, during my ethnographic study on natural gas drilling activism, I conducted twenty in-depth interviews. I invited people to speak with me who were the "key players" in the action—those whom I saw at the front of protests, leading grassroots efforts, and the most involved as activists. I also interviewed people in regulatory positions relevant to the study. Did I miss activists with other opinions? Probably. But I was clear about who my key informants were and that I was not trying to generalize to all activists. Instead, I was interested in what was happening in this particular place at that particular time.

We do, however, need to ensure that we are not myopic in our sampling. One of my doctoral students (Ellis 2020) conducted a study on graduate students who gave birth during their graduate programs to determine what supports and challenges they faced. She could have interviewed many of her friends, and friends of friends (she attended a women's university and potential subjects were readily available to her). She was concerned, however, that relying on her personal network would provide too narrow a focus. There was a high likelihood that people in her personal network had similar experiences to each other and that they already agreed with some of her own ideas about the problem. Instead, she recruited nationally and was able to get a diverse selection of women from all over the United States to participate. She also made a point to select a broad sample of women. She ended up with fifty interviews, which included students from both public and private universities; from unionized and non-unionized institutions; from single and married women; from heterosexual and homosexual women; from some international students; and from Asian, Black, Hispanic, and White women. This made for a more robust sample and allowed her to understand some of the differences within and between different groups of students, as well as finding commonalities in their experiences.

In most cases, it is not feasible for an entire population to be in your study. Unless the population is quite small, a researcher would be hard-pressed to interview everyone (in addition, some people might not want to participate). Because of this, we use a sample of a population instead. Table 3.2 outlines some of the most common sampling techniques used by researchers.

When reflecting on your sample, ask yourself if there are any people who should be in your study but who are being systematically excluded because of how you decided to conduct the research (Olson 2011: 54–55). For example, suppose you were interviewing cancer patients. Some might be able to meet you someplace and hold a traditional interview; others may be too weak to travel or to talk for a long time. Maybe you need to interview over the phone or internet, or keep the interview short to accommodate them.

TABLE 3.2 Common Types of Samples

Random sample	A random sample begins with a list of *all* the people in the population. The researcher then selects a random group from this list, such that every person on the list has an equal chance of being selected. Usually this is done with the help of a random number generator.
Convenience sampling	The researcher invites people to participate who are convenient to them. This can be people they already know, classmates, people in their church, or other groups they have relatively easy access to.
Purposive sampling	The researcher identifies and invites people with a particular characteristic the researcher is interested in to be part of the research. Perhaps they are part of an organization the researcher is studying or members of a particular identity category.
Snowball sampling	Asking people who have agreed to participate in the research if they know others who might be interested in participating, and then inviting those people to participate as well.

Funding

Many qualitative researchers argue there is no "cost" to their work because they do not need to invest in specialized equipment. While the biologists are buying fancy microscopes and the physicists are spending money on lasers, we don't need much in the way of scientific instrumentation. There is a cost to all research, however, even if that cost is simply one's time. Given all the demands on a researcher's time that have nothing to do with getting their own research done, funding can be crucial to the researcher's ability to complete their projects.

This section is based on my knowledge and experience with research funding in the United States. It is important to note that other countries handle research funding differently. However, international researchers may find some helpful tips here.

I discuss two different categories of funding sources—internal to your university and external to your university. By internal funding, I mean funding opportunities that your university provides for research. These may or may not be competitive. Some of the opportunities my university offers include travel grants and small grants (less than $1,000) that are not competitive (although there is a limited amount of money that can be given away each year). We also have a variety of competitive grants, ranging from $5,000 to $10,000, and equipment grants that can top $100,000. And we have student research grants, which include travel grants and research grants (up to $1,500). Your university probably has something similar, and they are well worth investigating.

By external grants, I mean any funding source not affiliated with your university. These may be government grants (federal, state, or local), funding from private foundations, or even direct donations (e.g., from alumni or corporations). These can range from a few hundred dollars up into the millions.

I hear two complaints when I advise qualitative researchers to write grants. The first is that they don't know what they would spend the money on if they got it. The second is that grant writing is time-consuming (especially if they don't end up getting funding) and that they simply can't spare the time.

Let's begin with what to spend the money on. Items to consider in your budget include the following:

- Buyout for a course and/or summer salary
- Student research assistants, postdocs
- Transcription costs
- Equipment—high-quality audio, video, photography
- Software—transcription, analysis
- Travel, for data collection and for conference presentations
- Editing and, in the case of books, indexing
- Workshops, writing retreats, and other training
- Publication costs for open access journals
- Participant incentives

Read the calls for proposals (CFPs) closely to make sure that they will pay for what you want them to pay for. Ensure that your work is a good fit and that you address all of their requirements in your application. If your university has a grants office or Office of Research and Sponsored Programs (ORSP), visit them as early as possible to get assistance. They know the grant regulations for your state, and there may be things related to your budget you are not aware of. For example, there are usually set costs for research assistants and postdocs that your university allows, and you can't forget about benefits if you are hiring people. Some grants, especially government contracts, allow for indirect costs (IDCs) at a certain percentage of the total grant (this can be high, so budget accordingly). IDCs are funds from the grant that go directly to your institution and not to you. They are intended to pay for things such as keeping the lights on and the air-conditioning going, for maintenance and custodial work in your building, and everything else that keeps the university running so that you can get your job done. If IDCs are allowable on your grant, work with your university's grants office to help you factor them into your budget. These have a set rate that you will have no control over.

Where do you begin to look for grants? In the United States, all federal grants are listed at https://www.grants.gov. For state, county, and city grants, your jurisdictions may have a central database, or you may have to look at the individual websites of the entity you are interested in. For example, in Texas, state agencies offer all sorts of grants, but you have to look at each agency's website to find them. For example, the Texas Department of Parks and Wildlife offers funding for all sorts of projects, but you need to go to the grants section of their website to find the calls for proposals. This means you need to spend some time figuring out which agencies might fund the type of work that you do. But also think broadly. Texas Parks and Wildlife funds creative and educational projects as well as biology and chemistry research. The following are other places to consider looking for grant funding:

Professional organizations in your discipline
Local governmental organizations
Foundations
Nonprofit organizations
Hospital systems
Businesses (both corporate and local)
Private individuals (including alumni)

As you look over these funding sources, it may occur to you that they have an agenda with regard to funding research. They do. Very few funders just fund "research." Some foundations will fund basic research, but for the most part when someone is putting up money, they are doing so because they are looking for answers to a problem they are interested in. In fact, their funding may be tied to a specific research question that they are hoping you will answer. Because of this, there is an ethical concern you must contend with. Do you want to study their research question? What will you do if you find something contrary to what the funder is looking for? Be clear and upfront about what the expectations are, both for you and for the funder.

Grant writing is an important part of your career as a professor. And increasingly, universities will require you to recoup some, if not all, of your salary from grants.

Generally, you will want to start off small and then build off of your previous successes. Or you can join a research team that has already had some success and build from there.

First, you must establish a clear research agenda. This begins in graduate school with your dissertation and other publications. A grant reviewer should be able to look at your vita and see that you have the background and experience to do the type of project that you are proposing. For instance, if you are proposing a study of injuries in volleyball players but the only publications you have are on kinesiology pedagogy, you probably won't get the grant. The funder wants to know that you—out of all the other applicants—are the best person for the job. So before you aim for the big dollars, you need to get some publications in your research area.

If you are a student, your university may have travel grants and dissertation or other student research grants. Apply for them. Professional organizations also tend to have dissertation grants, so try for those too. For faculty, apply for internal grants to help build your record. This serves several purposes. It gives you the time and funds to conduct a small project and publish an article or two from it. It shows future funders that your university supports your work and thinks that it is worth funding. It also helps you demonstrate that you can manage a grant. Once you are successful with an internal grant or two, begin applying for external grants. Each success you have sets you up for an even larger grant.

Let me give you an example. LaWanna is a graduate student interested in the experiences of people of color who have been admitted to in-patient psychiatric care due to mental illness. She wants to build her career off this topic. A possible trajectory for her could look as follows:

1. LaWanna works with her major professor and is the second author on an article on African Americans and mental health.
2. She applies for a dissertation grant through her discipline's national organization. Because LaWanna is a member of a minority group, she also applies for a minority student fellowship through the organization.
3. LaWanna receives the fellowship. She writes her dissertation on people of color who were previously hospitalized in an in-patient psychiatric facility. She conducts twenty in-depth interviews for her project.
4. While working on her dissertation, she applies for, and gets, a travel grant so that she can present her work at a national conference. She also writes two articles from her dissertation and gets them published. She and her advisor co-author another article on a related topic.
5. LaWanna graduates and accepts a position as an assistant professor at a university. When she takes the job, she negotiates for a start-up package that includes a laptop, software, and a course release her first year so that she can have time to work on her research.
6. LaWanna publishes a third article from her dissertation.

7. LaWanna applies for a $10,000 grant from her university. She uses the funds to hire a graduate research assistant. They hold several focus groups of families who have had a family member hospitalized in an in-patient psychiatric facility.
8. LaWanna publishes two papers from this project.
9. She would like to do a larger, ethnographic study in a mental health facility. She finds one that is willing to let her do her study there.
10. She applies for a federal mental health research grant and receives $75,000. She uses the funds for course buyouts and graduate research assistants. She gets the grant and spends the next year collecting data.
11. LaWanna again applies for internal funding from her university, this time to buy out a class so that she has time to write a book about her ethnography. She gets the funds and writes the book.
12. While working on the book, she secures a contract with a university press to publish the book.
13. The book is published. LaWanna receives tenure.
14. LaWanna decides she would like to open a center that conducts research on mental health issues and people of color. She applies for a $1.2 million federal grant to set up the center and receives it. She uses part of the funds to pay for her salary as the director of the center. She now directs the center half time and works in her department half time. She also negotiates with the university that a percentage of indirect funds for all grants that come out of the center are returned to the center's operating budget.
15. The center becomes a place for all researchers working on mental health issues at her university to converge. They write many more grants, publish many more papers, and eventually host an annual conference. LaWanna is promoted to full professor and is a nationally recognized expert on mental health issues and people of color. She is regularly invited to give keynote talks at conferences. She writes another book, this time directed at in-patient facilities and how they can improve the quality of care for people of color.

In this example, everything went well for our hypothetical scholar. I didn't want the narrative to get too long, but she would have had failures along the way. Everyone does. Some of those papers may have been rejected a few times before they were published. She probably applied for grants that she didn't get. The point, however, is to demonstrate how to keep a research agenda moving forward and build off of previous successes.

I mentioned at the beginning of this section that many people I talk to about grants say they don't have time to write them. I argue the opposite. You don't have the time to waste not writing them. As you could see in the example I just gave, at every point that LaWanna received funds, *she was able to get time*, either through buying out a course or paying other people to do some of the work for her. This is probably the most important thing you get from grant writing—the extra time to do your research and make a name for yourself.

Let's turn now to some basic tips for writing the narrative portion of your grant. In the narrative, you will explain what it is you want to do with the money, why your work is important, and why you are the best person for the job.

Remember that when asking for money, the organization will want to know how this project will, either directly or indirectly, benefit *it*. You may have a wonderful project, but why would this group want to support it?

Because of this, your audience is of utmost importance. When you write a journal article, you are writing for your peers. This may not be the case when writing a grant—your peers may not be the people reviewing it. Therefore, the narrative of your grant proposal should be written in accessible language. Envision your audience as educated people who may not be familiar with the details of your academic field or the work you are proposing. I will never forget reviewing a grant proposal for some nutritional research on blueberries. I could not understand what the researchers planned to do, nor could I figure out the point of their research, despite all of their charts and graphs and lengthy list of references. All I got from reading their proposal was that it had something to do with blueberries. I love blueberries. I did not recommend the project for funding.

Reviewers of large federal grants will expect to see well-documented methods and discussion of how you are going to disseminate the results. Other organizations may be less interested in the technical information about your methodology. It is helpful to speak with a program officer at the organization to find out how much detail they want. In addition, most funders provide examples of successful proposals on their websites. If they don't, contact the program officer and ask if you could see examples of proposals they have funded. Take the time to read several of them if you have access, and model yours after them.

This is not the time to try to impress people with a lot of jargon. You need the reviewers to understand what you will do with the money and why your project should matter to them. Generally, the grant exists because the funder either needs some information or wants to have some project completed and is looking to give money to someone who will get it done for them. Show them you are the person to do it.

In the United States, the trend in federal funding is to support multidisciplinary research teams rather than solo researchers. This is good for qualitative researchers; we can usually support quantitative work with contextual data, allowing us an entry point into all sorts of research projects. I recently received a $1.5 million National Science Foundation grant as a co-principal investigator (PI; one investigator among four). The grant is to get more women and underrepresented groups into biotechnology. That's not my field of interest, but the other PIs wanted to have focus groups of the students in the program, and they asked me to conduct them. Indeed, funders often require both quantitative and qualitative analysis to provide a more robust understanding of the phenomena of research. For example, you may find some colleagues who are proposing to conduct a large, nationally representative survey and would like to include in-depth interviews in their study. Surveys are often constructed after in-depth interviews are conducted—beginning with in-depth interviews can help survey researchers refine their questions. After the survey is completed, in-depth interviews can be used to follow up on any unexpected or surprising findings. In-depth interviews provide important contextual information for understanding the survey results.

The most important advice I can give you about grants, however, is to keep writing them. Get feedback from the reviewers when you receive a rejection. Work with your grants office to improve your grant. Attend a seminar or take a class in grant writing. Find a mentor who has been successful in grant writing to help you. It will be time-consuming on the front end, to be sure. But it will also pay off in the long term and be a boon to your career.

Evaluating Qualitative Research

As you probably have noticed, a researcher must make many decisions about the research before they begin collecting information. How do we know if we've done good work? Savin-Biden and Major (2013: 123) offer the following list of questions to continually refer to in order to ensure we are on the right track. We can use these to evaluate others' qualitative research:

Clear
- Is the topic of the research clearly identified?
- Is it a significant topic?
- Is the purpose of the research clearly articulated?

Adequate grounding
- Is the research connected to prior research?
- Does the researcher use prior research either before or after data collection in order to connect the work to prior knowledge?
- Does the researcher indicate how the research corresponds with or advances current knowledge?
- Is the research connected to theory?
- Is the study theoretically positioned?
- Is the theory clear, insightful, and appropriate?
- Is there an alternative theory that would be a better choice?
- Is the theory actually a theory?

Research question
- Is the central question (phenomenon, culture, event, or other) clearly described?
- Has the researcher identified a well-defined question?
- Is the question interesting and important?

Research tradition
- Is a tradition indicated and validated?
- Does the tradition match the question?
- Is the question interesting and important?

Site and sample
- Was the site of the study described?
- Were the participants a reasonable group to select?

- Were an appropriate number of participants selected?
- Were they selected in a reasonable way?
- Were sound measures used to ensure confidentiality?

Data
- What data were used?
- Were they clearly described?
- Are the data sources free from obvious bias?
- Are there potentially better sources of data?
- How were data collected?
- Were sufficient data collected to support rich thick description?
- Was sufficient time spent in the field?
- Were appropriate procedures used to record and transcribe data?

Data analysis
- How were data analyzed?
- Were the methods clearly described?
- Were the methods selected the best ones?
- Was the researcher systematic in the data analysis process?
- Did the data support the analysis?

Results
- Were the results communicated clearly and succinctly?
- Do the findings make sense?
- Do the results answer the questions?
- Were data cited effectively?
- Are participants represented fairly and sensitively in the report?
- Are the conclusions convincing?
- Were appropriate caveats indicated?
- Are there alternative explanations for the results?
- Were findings verified?

Rigor
- Were approaches to validity or trustworthiness described?
- Does the researcher provide a plan to minimize potential bias?
- Has the researcher given sufficient detail to determine whether findings or methods might be generalizable?

Overall
- Did the researcher articulate decisions throughout the process?
- Did the researcher provide good rationale for those decisions?
- Is the study of practical or theoretical importance?

A well-designed study will help you get quality results, so it is important that you take the time to think through what it is you plan to do and how you are going to do it. Before you begin, become intimately familiar with the literature on your topic. This will help you know what has already been done and help you narrow the focus of your own research. Consider also how this project supports your research agenda, and thereby your career advancement.

References

Barad, Karen. 2007. *Meeting the Universe Halfway: Quantum Physics and the Entanglement of Matter and Meaning.* Durham, NC: Duke University Press.

Ellis, Erin. 2020. "Giving Birth in the Ivory Tower: A Closer Look at the Unique Needs of Pregnant and Parenting Graduate Student Mothers." Doctoral dissertation.

Gullion, Jessica Smartt. 2015. *Fracking the Neighborhood: Reluctant Activists and Natural Gas Drilling.* Cambridge, MA: MIT Press.

Gullion, Jessica Smartt. 2018. *Diffractive Ethnography: Social Sciences in the Ontological Turn.* London: Routledge.

Olson, Karin. 2011. *Essentials of Qualitative Interviewing.* Walnut Creek, CA: Left Coast Press.

Savin-Biden, Maggi, and Claire Howell Major. 2013. *Qualitative Research: The Essential Guide to Theory and Practice.* New York: Routledge.

St. Pierre, Elizabeth Adams. 2013. "The Appearance of Data." *Cultural Studies ↔ Critical Methodologies* 13, no. 4: 223–227.

Further Reading

Cochrane Reviews. https://www.cochranelibrary.com.

Preferred Reporting Items for Systematic Reviews and Meta-Analysis (PRISMA). http://prisma-statement.org.

Discussion Questions

1. When should you conduct a literature review? Why?
2. How do you determine the parameters of a study (e.g., people, time, place)?

Active Learning

1. Search https://www.grants.gov for calls for proposals related to research you are interested in conducting.
2. Check the websites of professional organizations you belong to for student grants and fellowships. Apply to the ones you qualify for.
3. Write a research proposal.

Mindfulness Exercises

1. How important is it for you to get out of your comfort zone when conducting research?
2. What fears do you have about conducting research?

4

Reflexivity and Diffraction

Researchers bring their own backgrounds and identity characteristics with them when they conduct research, and these can influence how they approach their studies. In this chapter, we explore issues of objectivity and bias, reflexivity, and diffraction in order to understand how to use our personal standpoints as an advantage and not a hindrance to our work.

We begin this chapter with an invitation for researchers to consider their own standpoints—who they are and how their experiences have shaped them as a person—and how one's standpoint has an impact on their research. We do this so that we are conscious of our own personal filters and how they might influence what we see and hear and the choices we make during the course of our project. This includes (and encourages) deep self-reflection. We also have to consider the relationships between the researcher and those being researched and the dynamics of the researcher–participant relationship.

Who we are, our roles and identities, matter. We bring our own experiences, background, and pasts to our research. We all have (often unconscious) things hidden behind the curtain, so to speak, that influence us, from the initial spark of interest in a topic to completion of the project. Your experience, beliefs, background, and past influence the emergence of your research question and every decision you make afterward. Although some researchers argue that you can "bracket" your standpoint, holding who you are as a person at a distance and separating yourself from your research, that is not realistic. Who we are and what we believe is real and true influence how we see and understand the world.

An important task in *any* type of research (qualitative, quantitative, or other) is the practice of reflexivity, which we discuss below. Likewise, through the course of your research, you create an interference with the phenomenon you are investigating. You change as

Doing research changes the researcher and the participants.

Qualitative Research in Health and Illness. Jessica Smartt Gullion, Oxford University Press. © Oxford University Press 2024.
DOI: 10.1093/oso/9780190915988.003.0005

a person, your intervention in the phenomenon you researched had an influence on that phenomenon, and you shaped emanations from the encounter. This is called diffraction. In this chapter, we explore both.

I think it is prudent, however, to begin our discussion with objectivity. Objectivity is reified as a value in science, yet it is a simulacrum—there is no objectivity in research.

Objectivity

As noted earlier, one of the critiques of qualitative inquiry is that it lacks objectivity. Although it is true that qualitative research differs from positivism, even positivism suffers from errors of objectivity.

Objectivity has long been considered a cornerstone of science. To be objective, a researcher must suspend any personal beliefs and feelings about the work they are doing. This is opposed to bias, which occurs when the researcher has a specific agenda that they are trying to achieve and data are collected and/or "massaged" to bring about the desired result. Clearly, no ethical researcher wants to do that, no matter what research method they use.

Proponents of objectivity state that the researcher should be "hands off" and in no way influence or be influenced by the outcome of the research. Yet when we talk about qualitative methods such as co-constructed knowledge, qualitative researchers violate that definition. We are instruments in the data collection and analysis processes, never truly outside of what we are researching; however, I argue the same holds true for quantitative researchers. "Social scientists by definition think about and with the world in which we are enmeshed" (Gullion 2018: 36). As we think about and with the world, we influence it.

The problem with objectivity is that research is never untouched by human intervention. Strega and Brown (2015: 7) write,

> Every decision a researcher makes, from choices about topic and research site to the minutiae of relationships with participants to the means by which findings are disseminated, has political significance and therefore affects the social justice potential of our work.

Likewise, Bhattacharya and Kim (2018: 3) write, "When we try to understand a research phenomenon, we are in a hermeneutic situation in which we bring our prejudices with us. Therefore, we are inevitably standing inside it rather than detached from it, objectively looking in." And Barad (2007: 90–91) notes that "we do not uncover preexisting facts about independently existing things as if they exist frozen in time like little statues positioned in the world. Rather, we learn about phenomena—about specific material configurations of the world's becoming." And we are part of that phenomena. We are not, nor can we be, objective when we do any type of social science research. From inception of the project through publication, the researcher makes all kinds of decisions that could have been made differently, and therefore could have had an impact on the results.

To address the problem of objectivity, researchers practice what is known as reflexivity.

Reflexivity

Reflexivity involves interrogating your standpoint—your identities, your beliefs, and anything else that makes you *you*—and exploring how they influence your research. Gullion (2018: 85) writes,

> Reflexivity is a practice of identifying and interrogating the ways in which characteristics of the researcher's self influence their research. It is intentionally self-referential. The researcher considers how and in what ways their standpoint in the world has an impact on the relationships and processes of research.

Often, faculty note they can learn a lot about their students by what their students choose to conduct research on. That choice reflects something about them. As Denzin (2010: 24) has noted, "All inquiry reflects the standpoint of the inquirer." This is an important point for us to remember at all stages of the research process. We need to be conscious of who we are, what we believe, how we view reality, and so on, so that we are also conscious of how those factors interplay with our research projects.

Reflexivity involves interrogating your standpoints.

Our standpoint is a crucial component of our research because it is the lens through which we view the world yet cannot remove. To some extent, our standpoint influences what we see, what we decide is important, and how we understand the world. The trouble is that we may not be aware of how our standpoint influences our thoughts and actions. My standpoint as a middle-aged educated White woman is different from that of a high school senior with a brain tumor who is also a person of color. Although I may do my best to understand what it is like to be her (through practices of radical empathy), I cannot truly know, and it is possible that I will make incorrect assumptions based on my own standpoint.

Dorothy Smith's classic article, "Women's Perspective as a Radical Critique of Sociology" (1974) demonstrates how this happens. In the early 1970s, more women were finding their way into faculty positions. They discovered that the theories which purported to describe their lives did little to inform them; in fact, the people most often studied were White Anglo-Saxon men of means, relative to some subordinate other. The researcher was almost always a privileged White man. Although these men argued that their work was objective, the inclusion of women's perspectives demonstrated that their work was clouded by their standpoint—and would be, until women scholars had the opportunities to raise their voices and point out the problems with this work. Women then wrote new theories that were more aligned with women's experiences.

We all inhabit our own reality. This does not mean that our realities cannot overlap with others' realities, but we must remain cognizant that what is reality for one person is not necessarily the reality of another.

Unfortunately, this type of thinking encourages cries that there is no reality or that we live in a world of false facts and "fake news." Disinformation is used in such a manner by some politicians and others wishing to sway public opinion. This encourages anti-intellectualism, beliefs that all facts are simply a matter of opinion, and beliefs that all opinions are equal. We must guard against this misuse of the argument. As Davis (2008: 28) writes,

> Researchers must make their own value positions clear, including the so-called facts and ideological assumptions that they attach to these positions. Scholars must identify and analyze the values and claims to objective knowledge that organizes positions that are contrary to their own. In so doing they will show how these appeals to ideology and objective knowledge reflect a particular moral and historical standpoint.

As you interrogate your own standpoint in the world, consider how the following might have an impact on your research. Your:

- Race/ethnicity
- Gender
- Sexual preference
- Education level
- Social class
- Marital status
- Country of origin
- Native language
- Religion (or lack thereof)/spiritual beliefs

This list could go on and on. Once you've interrogated identity variables, you can ask yourself a host of additional questions:

- How do your own values and beliefs influence your research?
- How does your personal history influence your research?
- Why did you choose the topic you want to research?
- What led you to that topic?
- What assumptions do you hold about your subject matter?
- How do your various identities allow you to move through people and spaces of interest?
- How much of your research is about *you*?

As you go through this exercise, you might find that there are some topics you cannot study. For example, I know that I cannot study anything related to child abuse. My opinions are too strong, and I would never be able to control the impact of my standpoint on that research topic. I also know that immersing myself in that world would cause me trauma.

When practicing reflexivity, we consider not only our own backgrounds but also our impressions of and the standpoints of the research participants. What if you think a participant is sexy? An idiot? Racist? Sexist? Just plain creepy? What if you think they are better than you? Smarter than you? How will those impressions influence your interaction with them and, by association, the data that you collect from them?

We can easily misread people based on our standpoint. I found myself in a situation recently in which I quickly judged a participant and I had to go back and reflect on how my own stereotypes influenced the interaction. When I first met this woman and we had an initial, small-talk conversation, I categorized her in my head as a "wealthy wine mom"—someone who doesn't work outside the home, spends a lot of time driving her kids around to sporting events, and who drinks a lot of wine. Those things were all true about her. However, I later learned that she was an alcoholic, struggling to stop drinking, who had been severely physically and sexually abused as a child. She had been in and out of rehab centers a number of times due to her drinking and suicide attempts. She was in her second marriage and was wealthy at the time I met her, but her first marriage ended badly and at one point she and her child lived in her car. Had I not had an ongoing relationship with her, my initial impressions would have stuck, and I would have read and analyzed the transcript of our conversation very differently. I would have missed some of the most important parts of her story.

Whether or not we want to admit it, we categorize people we meet. We put them in a mental box. We want to know if they are safe for us to be around and if we are comfortable talking with them or spending time with them. We must always be aware of the judgments we make of people. It's natural to want to put people into a framework that we already know, but doing so can be detrimental to our research. Rather than feigning objectivity, we should acknowledge and interrogate our gut reactions to others.

As you get to know people better, the details of their lives spool out like Ariadne's thread. People are complex; it's bad research to prejudge our partici-

> Researchers should acknowledge and interrogate their perceptions of their research participants.

pants. When I reflected on my prejudgment of the woman mentioned previously, I realized that I had put her into a category of women I knew from my own child's sports activities— moms who are actively involved in their children's activities and who also often have wine in expensive insulated cups that they bring to their children's sporting events.

This also speaks to the drawbacks of one-time encounters with our participants. I got to know this woman over several weeks. If I had spoken to her once and left it at that, I never would have learned her backstory. I might have stuck to my initial impressions of her and missed the depth of her lived reality. I might have used that initial impression unconsciously while I was analyzing her interview, and it probably would have influenced my interpretations of what she told me.

There is much debate about whether or not the interviewer should "match" the participants' demographics. Some of this comes down to the study topic and how you think people will respond. As an example, I was recently part of a team studying how faculty respond to racism in the classroom. We had a long debate about who should conduct the focus group. The participants could have been of any racial/ethnic group, but given the population demographics, it was likely that most, if not all, of the participants would be White. We wanted to know how they would respond to questions about race, but would they be more likely to share their thoughts with a White interviewer or a person of color? Would they be more likely to censor themselves in the presence of a researcher with different social characteristics than them? Likewise, would the gender of the interviewer matter? Or the level of education? We debated having graduate students lead the focus group instead of a fellow faculty member. That raised issues of power. As an aside, this proved to be moot as we were unable to get faculty to participate.

It is possible that you will be working as part of a research team. The question of who will interact with participants is part of the study design. Will you do it, or will a member of your research team do it? The person who has contact with the participants can influence how they will respond to questions.

Most qualitative researchers now include some sort of reflexivity statement(s) in their writing, and they keep a reflexivity journal to work through these issues on paper. Unfortunately, this is not yet the norm for quantitative researchers (who clearly could be just as influenced by their standpoints as qualitative researchers). It is hoped that this will shift.

As you can see, when we really get into the details of qualitative research, things get tricky. However, the more we think through these issues, the better our study will be.

When reflexivity becomes the project in itself, the researcher may move to writing autoethnography. Many researchers, troubled by the various problems they see in social science, do just that. Autoethnographers use their own lives as data, and they critically explore their experiences as embedded in a larger context. For example, a charge nurse might write about her experiences in the job but also relate those experiences to larger issues of power in the hospital and power in the health care system. A psychologist working with autistic children could write about what that was like, while also providing a critical analysis of the ways in which neurodivergent children are labeled and treated, or how funding impacts the quality of care the children she worked with received, which then impacts quality of life as those children age out of the program.

Diffraction

In addition to practicing reflexivity—recognizing and understanding how our own standpoint impacts our research—we need to practice diffraction. This is a recognition of how we create and are shaped by our research. Whereas reflexivity is like a mirror reflecting on the researcher, diffraction explores the ways in which both the researcher and the phenomenon under research are changed in the course of a research project. Diffraction also invites us to consider intra-action with the material agents that are also part of the phenomena of interest.

Diffraction is involved in the process of co-constructing knowledge. In my 2018 book, *Diffractive Ethnography: Social Sciences in the Ontological Turn*, I explored how we might do social science that is inclusive of nonhumans—that gives nonhumans agential capacity. I took the stance articulated by Barad (2007: 66) that "what is needed is a robust account of the materialization of *all* bodies—'human' and 'nonhuman'—including the agential contributions of all material forces (both 'social' and 'natural')."

Both reflection and diffraction are ways of seeing. They describe optics. With reflection, one sees the reversed image of oneself. With diffraction, one sees the ways one is changed through intra-action with another agent. This area of change is known as an interference pattern, and it is ripe for analysis. We interfere with a phenomenon when we study it. We interfere with people's lives, like two waves intermingling with each other, creating a new wave pattern in their wake.

Whereas with reflexivity, a researcher interrogates how their standpoint and identity impact their research, diffraction asks a researcher to interrogate how they and the phenomena they research are changed by the act of research, in a way that creates something new.

The notion of diffraction comes from physics. Previously, I mentioned waves and how we act like waves when we intra-act in our research. To understand diffraction, let's think about waves in the ocean and the ways that they crash into each other, overlap, combine, dissipate. Waves are not "things"; they are disturbances in water or air or other medium. "When waves encounter an obstruction, they bend and spread, move and combine. Interference patterns happen where waves overlap and diffract" (Gullion 2018: 115). What if the researcher is a "wave," as are the things and people they encounter? That encounter diffracts. It is a disturbance that leaves all of the entities involved changed. This is not a metaphor but, rather, a phenomenon that actually happens.

Even more interesting is the notion of entanglement—what happens when the waves meet. "When we talk about entanglement, we are not saying things are mixed together, or that they are in a causal relationship, but rather that they are *intertwined at the quantum level*" (Gullion 2018: 117). Researchers and the subjects and objects of research become entangled during the research process. They connect, and something new emerges.

Qualitative researchers have become attached to reflexivity as a way to position their standpoint and be transparent about the relationship between their standpoint and their scholarly work. Reflexivity has, however, come under some criticism as to whether or not it does anything to *enhance* research. Haraway (cited in Barad 2014: 172) argues that "diffraction does not produce 'the same' displaced, as reflection and refraction do. Diffraction is a mapping of interference, not of replication, reflection, or reproduction." She argues that reflexivity repeats (reflects) the same, like a mirror, whereas diffraction creates something new.

Thus, diffraction is an invitation for social scientists to map interference as a different way of knowing relative to replication, reflection, or reproduction (Gullion 2018). Barad (2007: 90) challenges us to take a critical approach by asking "which differences matter, how they matter, and for whom." Rather than acknowledging and describing differences between us and our participants (as we might do reflexively), she invites us to consider power effects and other dynamics that shape the phenomena we are studying.

"Rather than an optics of reflection—spending our time describing people and the things they do—we shift to an optics of diffraction—we ask questions about how assemblages work and how boundaries are configured and reconfigured" (Gullion 2018: 118). Researchers are not passive receptacles of data who objectively analyze them. Rather, we are an active part of a process, a world-making. We are an agential creative force—observing, interacting, changing—but we are not the only agential creative force in the research. Using this sort of approach, ontologically there is no hierarchy between subject and object in the world-making; rather, there are intra-actions between actants.

Barad (2007) uses what she calls a diffractive reading to emphasize how waves of knowledges intra-act. She advocates practices "of reading insights through one another in attending to and responding to the details and specificities of relations of difference and how they matter" (p. 71). Kirby (2011: x) extends this idea of reading to a multitude of entities: "The 'texts' of seemingly primeval organisms, or even a supposedly inanimate and lifeless entity such as a photon, become subjects of cognitive and agential entanglement and observational intention." As we engage in diffraction, we turn our attention away from identity and meaning toward an exploration of dynamic unfoldings and processes of change.

> Researchers are not passive receptacles of data who objectively analyze them.

Many considerations happen behind the scenes when we conduct research, and we have yet to discuss how to collect and analyze data (don't worry, that's coming up next). Good research involves more than just asking people questions and reporting what they said. It involves a deep dive into the philosophical, ethical, ontological, and epistemological orientations in which our research happens. Without delving into these aspects of research, our results are superficial and pedestrian, and we may be missing some of the most important, and interesting, information about our projects.

References

Barad, Karen. 2007. *Meeting the Universe Halfway: Quantum Physics and the Entanglement of Matter and Meaning*. Durham, NC: Duke University Press.

Barad, Karen. 2014. "Diffracting Diffraction: Cutting Together-Apart." *Parallax* 20, no. 3: 168–187.

Bhattacharya, Kakali, and Jeong-Hee Kim. 2018. "Reworking Prejudice in Qualitative Inquiry with Gadamer and De/Colonizing Onto-Epistemologies." *Qualitative Inquiry* 24, no. 3: 1–10.

Davis, Charlotte Aull. 2008. *Reflexive Ethnography: A Guide to Researching Selves and Others*, 2nd ed. New York: Routledge.

Denzin, Norman. K. 2010. *The Qualitative Manifesto: A Call to Arms*. Walnut Creek, CA: Left Coast Press.

Gullion, Jessica Smartt. 2018. *Diffractive Ethnography: Social Sciences in the Ontological Turn*. London: Routledge.

Kirby, Vicki. 2011. *Quantum Anthropologies: Life at Large*. Durham NC: Duke University Press.

Smith, Dorothy E. 1974. "Women's Perspective as a Radical Critique of Sociology." *Sociological Inquiry* 44, no. 1: 7–13.

Strega, Susan, and Leslie Brown. 2015. *Research as Resistance: Revisiting Critical, Indigenous, and Anti-Oppressive Approaches*, 2nd ed. Toronto: Canadian Scholars' Press.

Further Reading

Barad, Karen. 2007. *Meeting the Universe Halfway: Quantum Physics and the Entanglement of Matter and Meaning*. Durham, NC: Duke University Press.

Gullion, Jessica Smartt. 2018. *Diffractive Ethnography*. London: Routledge.

Haraway, Dona. 2016. *Staying with the Trouble: Making Kin in the Chthulucene*. Durham, NC: Duke University Press.

Discussion Questions

1. Why is objectivity such a contested issue in science? Do researchers need to be objective? Why?
2. How does a researcher's standpoint impact their research?
3. How might a researcher practice both reflexivity and diffraction?

Active Learning

1. Read three journal articles on a topic that interests you. Does the researcher provide any type of reflexivity/diffraction statements? If yes, how does that influence your opinion of the quality of the research? If no, do you think that missing information could change your opinion of the quality of the research?
2. Keep a log of the assumptions you have as you interact with people over the next week. Write about the assumptions and why you hold them.

Mindfulness Exercises

1. How might your identity characteristics (race, gender, etc.) influence your research?
2. What assumptions do you hold about your area of scholarly interest?

PART II

Collecting Empirical Materials

5

Interviewing

Interviewing is the cornerstone of most qualitative research. Good interviewing is a skill that we can develop. In this chapter, we explore how to conduct interviews, different types of interviews, how to create a questionnaire, and tips for becoming a better interviewer.

Interviewing is arguably the most common research method used in qualitative inquiry; we ask people questions and they answer them, and through that interaction, we learn about a phenomena of interest. This conversation is (or at least should be) largely one-sided, with the participant doing the majority of the talking. Our job as interviewers is to listen and to guide the conversation where we want it to go.

A questionnaire is a list of questions and prompts that are asked during an interview.

What Makes for a Good Interview?

In speaking about being interviewed, Le Guin and Naimon (2018: 5) wrote, "The good interview is like a good badminton rally: You know right away that the two of you can keep that birdie in the air, and all you have to do is watch it fly." It's an exchange, where the interviewer and participant build a narrative together about the phenomena of interest. As Ellingson (2017: 103) writes, interviews are "mutual performances of self between interviewer and interviewee [that] create intersubjective meanings." And Morris (2015: 3) writes that

> in essence, [an in-depth interview] involves a researcher asking questions and following up on the responses of the interviewee in an endeavor to extract as much information as possible from a person (the interviewee) who has expertise on the topic/s the interviewer is interested in.

Qualitative Research in Health and Illness. Jessica Smartt Gullion, Oxford University Press. © Oxford University Press 2024.
DOI: 10.1093/oso/9780190915988.003.0006

During the course of the interview, a story is constructed about the phenomena of interest. This is not to suggest that you are creating a fiction. Rather, you and the participant have a conversation that builds a narrative in response to your research question.

In the interview, you and the participant co-create knowledge during your discussion. "Qualitative methodologists consider interviews to be active; that is, two (or more) participants generate meanings within the encounter, through verbal and nonverbal communication, framing interviewing as a co-construction within a specific context," Ellingson (2017: 102) writes.

Types of Interviews

Most textbooks identify three major types of interviews: structured, semistructured, and unstructured. During a structured interview, the interviewer uses a standardized set of questions and follows the questionnaire without deviation. The idea behind this practice is that interviews can better be compared across the group. An example of this type of interviewing is the U.S. census. Interviewers must ask the questions exactly as they are written and are not allowed to add prompts or other explanation outside of the written questionnaire.

This technique is particularly useful in large research projects with multiple interviewers. There is a standardization such that the researcher can make comparisons between people. One concern about this type of interviewing, however, is that the interviewer may not explain the questions beyond how they are written. If a participant asks, for example, what a particular term means, all the interviewer can do is reread the question.

In a semistructured interview, the researcher has a list of questions to ask but has flexibility to deviate from those questions. This is the most common type of interview done by qualitative researchers. The interviewer may prompt, rephrase questions, and follow unexpected lines of conversation, while still ensuring they capture a specific set of information. The questionnaire in this case is a guiding document without the rigidity of a structured interview.

An unstructured interview typically does not have a questionnaire, and it is conversational in style. The researcher usually has some idea of what they would like to discuss but otherwise leaves the interview open for a more natural conversation. When I conducted research on fracking, this was the approach I took. My opening question was, How did you get involved in fracking? Then I just let the participant talk. The interview proceeded as a conversation, with me engaging in deep listening and following up with questions about things the participant said. This is a good technique for capturing narratives, but it is difficult, if not impossible, to compare interviews from person to person.

A fourth type of interviewing is oral history. In this type of interview, the researcher explores key moments in the person's life or moments that are related to a specific historical event. For example, you might imagine asking people what they did early in the COVID-19 pandemic. This captures facets of history that would be missed by examining the media and other reports of what happened. Oral histories may be structured, semistructured, or unstructured, but they are centered around a historical event. National Public Radio's Story Corps project[1] is an excellent example of oral history. Interviews from oral history projects are often archived so that other researchers may access and use them.

To decide which type of interview to use, it's important to think through what you would like the information to look like when it is time for analysis. Do you want to know every person's experience so that you can compare and contrast them? Are you looking for stories and different perspectives about a particular subject? Will there be more than one person conducting interviews? Or will someone besides you conduct the interviews? Many researchers choose the semistructured interview for its flexibility and consistency, but there are times when one would want to use the other types of interviews. Some participants welcome a structured interview. They expect you to sit in front of them with your tape recorder and ask them questions from a list you have on paper. The reality, however, is that this is not the best way to talk in depth with people about their experiences; they are less likely to relax and expound on the subject.

I've found that no matter the type of interview I conduct, the more conversational I can be, the richer the data that I collect. To get to that conversational space, you must know your interview tool. Memorize it. Practice with people you know before you begin the interviews for your research. If you robotically move through the questions (e.g., "Question number two asks . . ."), you will tend to get shorter answers and might miss opportunities to dig deeper into what the participant has said. This is also the case if you are constantly thinking about what you will ask next rather than giving the participant all of your attention.

Writing Questions

The questions you choose to ask of your participants should be guided by your research question. When I was a beginning researcher, I conducted a study on how likely it would be for school nurses to volunteer to help during a bioterrorism attack (Gullion 2004). I used a previously validated scale on volunteerism and another on preparedness for a bioterrorist attack. Although I got some great information, I never actually asked the question, Would you volunteer during a bioterrorist attack? With that oversight, I'm frankly surprised the study was published.

You should have a clear research question in mind before you start to write your questionnaire. Use that research question to structure the questionnaire. If you need to, straight out ask your research question. I should have done that with my bioterrorism project, instead of dancing around the answer I wanted to know.

Let's look at an example. Suppose your research question is the following: How do infection control professionals limit hospital-acquired infections? Let's build a questionnaire about that.

---

1. https://www.npr.org/series/4516989/storycorps.

Research Question: How do infection control professionals limit hospital-acquired infections?

Q1	How long have you worked in infection control?	This is an easy question that helps build rapport.
Q2	What are some of the things you do to limit hospital-acquired infections in your facility?	This question relates specifically to your research question.
Prompts	Can you tell me more about that? Can you give me an example?	The prompts may or may not be needed, but they are there to remind the interviewer to use them if needed.
Q3	Can you tell me about hospital-acquired infections at your facility?	This may be sensitive. They may not want to talk about this if there are many infections.
Q4	What do you think contributes to this?	This question works for both positive and negative answers to the previous question.
Q5	What sorts of handwashing campaigns do you do?	This question comes from the literature as a facet of an infection control professional's work.
Prompt	How do people respond to those campaigns?	This is a follow-up to the previous question.

These are probably not all the questions you would need; I just want you to have an idea of what the questionnaire might look like for that topic. Additional questions would be tied to the literature, or they might follow a path opened up during the discussion. Suppose for the question, "What sorts of handwashing campaigns do you do?" the participant answered, "I am limited by what I can do by the head nurse." You could follow up with, "How so?" rather than simply moving to the next question. If you accept that response without prompting further, you will probably miss some important information about your research question.

If you get stuck and have trouble coming up with questions, you can find ideas in the literature. What have other investigators asked about this topic? If their questions are useful, use them (and attribute them appropriately when you write up your results).

In order to maximize responses from your participants, your questions should be open-ended. This means that you shouldn't ask questions that the participant can respond to with single words (yes/no) or short phrases unless absolutely necessary. I've also heard that good interviews should avoid "why" questions because people can feel personally attacked, as if they have to justify their actions. Instead, rephrase those to "how" questions. For example,

Why did you major in kinesiology?
How did you decide to major in kinesiology?

The "why" question can put the participant on the defensive, whereas the "how" question gives them a chance to explain without judgment.

You should also avoid asking double-barreled questions. These are questions that are really two questions rolled into one. For example, don't ask, "How did you become a nursing major and wind up at this university?" Instead, make that into two separate questions: "How did you become a nursing major? How did you wind up at this university?" The reason for avoiding this type of question is that most people will not remember the whole question as they start to answer it. Rather than getting a confused, half-answer, just ask two questions.

It's also important that you avoid leading questions—questions to which a reasonable person would answer the way you wanted them to. We see this often in political polls that are sponsored by a particular candidate. Leading questions are written in such a way that it would be awkward for the participant to reply counter to the main point of the question. Any question that starts with "Don't you agree with . . ." or "Isn't it true that . . ." are signs of leading questions. The following example is from a survey conducted by the Trump campaign for the 2020 U.S. presidential election: "Do you think the current strength of the American economy will help President Trump's chances of reelection?"[2] It is leading because it includes the assumption that the current American economy is strong and that it is so because of Trump's previous actions; it leads the respondent to answer yes. An answer of no would not make much sense, even if the respondent had no intention of voting for Trump. Questions such as this provide biased data that are reported to the public, often to mislead people or mischaracterize people's beliefs.

If you are not using a structured questionnaire, you can use probes to encourage a participant to give more information. Examples of probes include phrases such as "Tell me more about that" or "Would you clarify what you mean by that?" Probing questions are especially helpful when the participant is not saying much or is only giving brief answers to your questions. Remember that this is "in-depth" interviewing. Explore the subject in depth with your participant.

In addition to writing good questions, think about the order in which you put them. What will make for a more natural conversation? Whereas in survey research demographics are typically asked at the end, in an interview, asking such questions first can help break the ice. You can also start with some background questions. For example, you could start with "How did you get involved with this?" It's a neutral question that can get the person talking.

If you plan on asking sensitive questions, don't jump right in. Find ways to ease into the subject so that your participant feels more comfortable talking to you. As you might imagine, some topics are more sensitive than others, and researchers need to be prepared for how to study them. Asking a participant to tell you about their participation in a recreational activity, for example, is much less sensitive than asking them to tell you about the time they were sexually assaulted.

From a relational ethics perspective, you should never blindside your participant with questions about sensitive issues. If you're studying sexual assault, for example, that information should be in the consent form. This is what informed consent is all about. The participant should come into the interview knowing that will be a topic of conversation so they can be prepared to discuss it. During an interview, remind your participant that they can skip any question they don't want to answer or that they can take a break from or stop the interview without repercussions. If you find a participant is having difficultly, you might want to ask a more neutral question and circle back to the more sensitive question later.

2. https://www.donaldjtrump.com/landing/the-official-2020-strategy-survey.

This both gives them a break and helps build rapport so they are more comfortable with the conversation (rapport is further discussed later in this chapter).

Once you have constructed your questionnaire, take the time to pretest the tool. I usually find a few people and ask them to pretend that they are part of the group I'm interviewing (or, even better, ask members of the target group who will not take part in the study), and then we have mock interviews. When we're done, I ask for their input about how they thought the interview went. As you pretest your instrument, think about the following:

Did you stumble on the wording of any of the questions?
Did the respondent understand all of the questions?
Did you have to clarify anything as you went?
Did the order of the questions make sense?
Did the order of the questions facilitate a conversation?
Did any of the questions seem redundant or that you didn't really need?
Did you get the information you needed to respond to your research question?
Was there any information you wanted but didn't get?
Did any of the questions lead the respondent off track from the overall discussion?
How long was the interview?
Did the respondent get bored during the interview?
Did you get bored during the interview?

This helps you refine your questions and get a feel for how much time an interview will likely take.

I generally aim for an hour-long interview, plus or minus fifteen minutes. Some people will want to talk for much longer, which is fine with me. I am suspicious of interviews less than forty-five minutes. Unless the issue is very narrow, it's unlikely that an interview shorter than that will get enough information to address the research question. On the other hand, in an interview that runs too long, the participant may become fatigued or get bored with the process. I do find, however, that people like to talk about themselves and their experiences, and often they will talk as long as you let them. Because of this, part of your job as the interviewer is to keep the conversation on topic. Depending on how much information I am looking for, I may interview the person more than once or contact them later for clarification of something they said.

"Most interviews start off slowly, all have peaks and valleys, and sometimes the most enlightening statements and useful responses are made following a 'clearinghouse' question at the end of the interview," Ellingson (2017: 104) writes. That clearinghouse question is usually something such as "Is there anything else you would like to say?" or "Is there anything we missed that we should talk about?" This is always the last question I ask.

I also make a point to leave the recorder running until the participant and I part. I do not hide that I am doing so; I want them to know it is still recording. Many times when you are leaving, the participant will remember something or say something off the cuff that is important to your study.

While we are conducting interviews, another consideration is the impact of power differentials between the interviewer and the participant. Power issues can also have a significant influence on your research. Morris (2015: 4) writes about four different power issues that researchers should consider in conducting interviews:

1. The person being interviewed is expected to "open up" and divulge information to the interviewer despite the fact that in almost all cases the latter is a stranger and is not expected to disclose much about themself.
2. The interview often involves the asking of questions that are personal and which the interviewee may have never discussed with anybody or even thought about.
3. The interviewer is likely never to see the interviewee again.
4. The interviewer is usually in control of the interaction and decides whether the questions have been satisfactorily answered and when the interview should conclude.

If we think about these concerns while constructing our questionnaire, we can help mitigate some of them. We can do the same during the interview. Think about how power is being used, and try to minimize the power differential between you and the participant.

Recruiting

Your institutional review board (IRB) will want to know how you will recruit participants to take part in your study, and this is something you will want to consider before you begin the research.

Do you have access to the group you want to study? Perhaps you already know some people in the study population. This can be tricky; although it is convenient to start your interviews with people you know, you need to ensure that they don't feel obligated (i.e., coerced) to take part in the study.

There are all sorts of ways to recruit potential participants. One way is to find a gatekeeper who will help you get in contact with people in your study population. For example, suppose you were interested in studying the use of needle exchange programs. The director of such a program is a gatekeeper who can help you access that population. You can post fliers on bulletin boards or virtually in online special interest groups (be sure you have the moderator's permission before doing so). You can post a flier on your own social media and ask others to share it. If you are a member of an organization related to the topic, the organization may be willing to send your information to their membership.

Go places where the type of people you'd like to interview hang out. When I did my ethnography on fracking, I went to city council and town hall meetings and introduced myself to people and told them about my research. That helped me identify potential participants and tell them about what I was doing. For an ethnography I am currently working on about cheerleading, I've spent a lot of time in gyms, at cheer competitions, and at football games. Spending time in the spaces potential participants inhabit is a great way to recruit (just be sure that it is ok for you to be there).

Once you begin interviewing, you can use a process called snowball sampling. This is when you ask the person you've interviewed to give your contact information to anyone they know who might be interested in participating in your study. Snowball sampling is a great way to find participants you might otherwise not have access to. One concern with snowball sampling, however, is homogeneity. Because the participants know each other, there is a likelihood that they hold similar beliefs or that they have had similar experiences. Snowball sampling can limit the diversity of participants, so you should not rely on snowball sampling exclusively.

Interviewing Logistics

Let's go through the basic steps that take place during an interview:

1. Identify a participant. Inform the participant what the study is about.
2. Decide together where and when you will meet to conduct the interview (even if this is online).
3. When you both arrive, thank the participant for attending the interview.
4. Remind the participant why you are both there: that you are a researcher and what you are conducting research on.
5. Review the consent form with them. Give them time to read it, and then ask them if they have any questions. Depending on their literacy level, you may want to read it to them. Make sure they sign the form. They give you the signed form and then you give them a blank form they may keep for their own records. The consent form should have both your contact information and information about how to contact your IRB if they have any concerns about your research.
6. Tell them they can stop the interview at any time without penalty, and they can skip any question if they would like to do so.
7. Ask if they have any questions.
8. Ask if it is ok to record them. If they say yes, turn on the recorder. If they say no, ask if you can take notes. In most cases, you will want to record the interview for later transcription. Recording also allows you to pay attention to the conversation without scrambling to take detailed notes about what the participant says.
9. Ask them if they understand the conversation is for research and if they consent to participating, so you have a recording of their consent.
10. Ask the first question. This should be nonthreatening to build rapport.
11. Carry on through your questions.
12. Be mindful of the participant's body language. Becoming emotional about what they are talking about is normal and common in research. You may be asking about something that is painful for them to talk about. However, if they show signs of significant distress, retraumatization, or dissociation, offer them a break and skip to a nonthreatening question. If you need to end the interview to protect their mental health, do so. Their well-being is more important than your getting the interview.

13. Once you have finished asking your questions, ask them if there is anything they didn't talk about that they think you need to know.
14. Thank them for taking the time to participate.
15. As soon as possible after the interview, write field notes. Write as much as you can remember about the interview, especially about nonverbal communication, your thoughts about how it went, and any other information you think is important.

Where to Interview

There are several considerations researchers should take into account when identifying a place to conduct a face-to-face interview. I usually ask participants where they would like to meet and, if reasonable, I meet them there.

Typically, one's university office is a terrible place to conduct interviews. The office is ripe with power signifiers, not to mention that if a participant isn't a member of the academic community, they will have to navigate the university's parking and find the location on campus. The obvious power differential will likely impact the interview. Instead, it is better to find a location in which *both* you and your participants feel safe and at ease.

The location should be relatively free of background noise and should afford the participant privacy. I often conduct interviews at coffee shops or restaurants during non-peak hours; however, both background noise and privacy can be problematic. I once conducted an interview outside during the summer at a snow cone stand at a participant's request. It was unbearably hot, there were numerous bees attracted to the snow cone syrup, and there was noise of children playing and passing cars. The participant chose the location intentionally—it was across the street from a fracking operation and they wanted me to experience the noise and fumes as residents experience them. I did. My mind was less focused on the interview than it should have been, however, and it was difficult to transcribe the interview given the level of background noise.

Some participants will want to be interviewed in their homes. If this is the case, you should be mindful of your own safety. In some cases, you may feel at ease with this; in others, you may not. Use your judgment and make sure you don't end up in a situation that you are not comfortable with.

Wherever you and your participant decide to conduct the interview, for your own safety, tell someone where you are going. Consider turning on the location service on your phone so that someone knows where you are. My family and I have an app on our phones with a map that shows where each of us is when our phones' location service is turned on. No one outside our family has access to it. Bear in mind too that you have the right to end the interview and leave, just as your participants do.

For a variety of reasons, you may decide to conduct the interview over the phone or using a video conferencing service. During the COVID-19 pandemic, before the vaccine was available, my university's IRB decided that for safety, all interviews had to be conducted over a secure video conferencing platform unless there were compelling reasons that was not feasible. If you and your participant choose this route, make sure that the technology is secure (e.g., use a password to get into the meeting). Also ensure that both you and your participant are mindful of privacy in your surroundings. On your end, that means that no one else should be able to hear you conduct the interview (e.g., office mates or family members if you are working from home).

Interviews do not have to be face-to-face. Be aware, however, of how the technology you use influences your interview, and determine what is the best technique for your particular participants. For example, I know from texting my kids and watching how they text their friends that they like to communicate over text, but I've found that I should only text one thought at a time if I'm going to interview this way. Two questions in one text, or even a long text, can result in confusion or in one question being missed.

Any communication that does not involve seeing the other person means you will lose the benefit of observing body language and nonverbal cues. I suspect many of us have had the experience of not realizing someone was being sarcastic or funny online and interpreted their words differently from how they meant it. The same can happen in your interviews. If you are unsure about the intent of a response (and you are not using a structured interview), ask for clarification.

Building Rapport

Rapport involves how comfortable the participant is when speaking with you. The more comfortable they are, the better the interview tends to go. We give signals to others, whether consciously or not, that help them be at ease with us. Being mindful of those signals will go a long way to establishing rapport.

While I was working on my natural gas ethnography, I set up an appointment with a young woman (she was in her early 20s) who had breast cancer that she believed resulted from the chemicals she had been exposed to from the gas well that was right next to her house. We met at a restaurant that she chose for an interview—a deli in her neighborhood.

> Rapport involves how comfortable the participant is when speaking with you.

We both ordered sandwiches and drinks, and I reviewed the project with her and we went over the consent form. She said she understood what we were doing and that she wanted to take part, and she signed the consent form. And then she sat quietly.

We could not connect. Every question I asked her was met with brief, stilted answers. I tried, but I couldn't get her to open up. I was disappointed because I really wanted to get her story, but sometimes this happens—an interview just doesn't work out.

I decided to give up and just enjoy my sandwich, which was quite good. I started talking about my kids (we had being mothers in common), not to get her to talk but more to fill the awkward silence. I told her about how the school that my children attended had two natural gas wells on the property and how that worried me for their health. I was torn, however, because it was a fantastic school and they loved being there. They had many friends and were both socially active, and I did not want to pull them out and find someplace else to send them. I talked about how it shouldn't be so difficult to find both good and safe education for one's children.

She blossomed. It was like I was sitting with a new person. Our children turned out to be our point of connection. She talked about her kids, and we had a great conversation about being mothers and raising kids around gas drilling. And after a while, without my prompting, she told me her own story, about getting breast cancer and going through treatments, and about the fact that there was a group of young mothers in her neighborhood who all had breast cancer and a cluster of children with leukemia—so many that someone started a support group at the elementary school.

I had built rapport with her without realizing what I was doing.

Let's look at another example of how to use rapport and how to probe for richer data. This comes from a project that one of my students conducted. For context, the interviewer was a Black PhD student who was also an Army veteran who retried at a high rank. The participant was an early career, Black, active-duty soldier. Also for context, the interviewer was a large man, approximately six feet four inches and muscular.

Interviewer: Let's talk about race in the military. Have you seen anything you would describe as racist since you've been enlisted?
Participant: No, sir.

Now, first off, we have to acknowledge that asking a yes or no question in a qualitative interview is a bad practice. It doesn't invite a participant to talk. Rather, like the example above, it allows the participant to respond with brief answers. There was also a power issue— my student's rank when he was in the military was higher than that of the person he was interviewing, and he is a big, intimidating guy. The interviewer could have stopped here and moved on to his next question. Had he done so in all of his interviews, he might have concluded that racism isn't an issue in the military. But instead, the researcher went off script and said the following:

Interviewer: Man. I remember my first week in boot camp. There was this White guy who kept calling me Big Boy. I mean, I'm big, no lie.
Participant: [Laughs]
Interviewer: But man he kept on with it. Big Boy! He'd shout it at me. And I'm like, I ain't your Boy, son.
Participant: [Laughs] This one guy, he asked if I knew any gangsters, if I was in a gang. You think they'd let me enlist if I was in a gang? Man, I grew up in rural Kansas. All I know about gangbangers is from TV and music.

The conversation continued from here.

Rapport involves making a connection with the other person, not in a manipulative way but, rather, in an authentic way. Sometimes that means we may share points of commonality with them. We humanize and normalize the exchange so that the participant is comfortable speaking with us.

To build rapport, another consideration is your own presentation of self. Although I'm not going to change my personality, I do wear clothing that more closely matches that of my participants. If I am interviewing rural veterinarians, I am coming to the interview in jeans and boots. If I am interviewing college students, I am going to wear casual clothing, maybe a T-shirt and jeans and flats. If I am interviewing physicians, I have found it best to wear business attire—a skirt and jacket. People judge you on how you look, and looking more like them is one way to help build rapport. Wearing a business suit to interview undergraduate students gives off a visible power signal at first sight. Instead, the goal is to minimize the power differences while still being true to ourselves.

Remember too that as an academic who works in the health field, topics you are comfortable with may be uncomfortable for your participants to discuss. Not long ago, I had a conversation with a health care professional who explained to me how doctors remove foreign objects that have become "lost" in people's anal cavities. This is not a conversation everyone would be comfortable having.

Deep Listening

"An individual's story is always only that which the listener makes of it," Arndt (2017: 95) writes. Deep listening is one facet of respect for persons. We give the participant our full attention, and we listen without thinking about what we are going to say next. This is not easy. Most of the time, we only half listen to people, while composing what we plan to say next in our heads. Don't do this. Your questionnaire is partly there so that you don't have to think about what you will say next—it's written down in front of you.

I typically advise people not to take notes during an interview unless the participant does not consent to recording. You are not fully listening when you are trying to write down what your participant is saying. Let the recorder do its job while you actively participate in the conversation. Later, you can transcribe the recording and get on paper exactly what was said. If you are worried about the technology failing and losing the interview, use two recording devices.

Part of deep listening involves paying attention to the participant's body language. We tend to focus on the words people say and overlook everything else. Yet, most of our communication with others happens through nonverbal communication (Ellingson 2017). Observe their body language and facial expressions. Do they seem bored? Upset? Make adjustments if needed. Deep listening is an embodied experience (Ellingson 2017).

Let's examine deep listening closer with an example. Being embodied means that you are aware of your own bodily reactions and those of your participant both during and immediately after the interview. When the interview has ended, include reflection on this in your field notes. Also, as you transcribe the interview, make notes to yourself about what the two of you were doing at different moments. Here's an example transcript that includes embodied reactions (where "I" is the interviewer and "P" is the participant):

I: How did you find out you had breast cancer?

This was a question from my questionnaire. The rest of the conversation was not on my questionnaire, but rather an emerging conversation between the two of us.

P: She [the doctor] didn't say, "you have cancer."

She paused here and then her eyes welled up.

P: It was after my sonogram, and the technician told me to stay there, on the exam table. She [the doctor] came in and handed me her business card, and said, "My cell phone number is on the back, you can use it when you need to."

She stopped talking here and started crying. I handed her a napkin and kept silent.

P: Then she said "you're young and healthy, you will get through this."

She had kind of a sad smile on her face after she said this.

I: But she still hadn't said the word cancer?

I remember thinking this was an odd behavior of the doctor, but maybe the doctor was trying to lessen the blow? While showing compassion by giving her the cell phone number?

P: No.

She said this firmly, still sounding upset.

I: When did someone say cancer?

Here, I'm trying to get the original question answered.

P: After I got dressed, the nurse took me into the doctor's office. That's when we talked about cancer. But I knew when she handed me her card.

She was in the sonogram room having a sonogram of her breast when the doctor gave her the card. Which means she wasn't fully dressed and was in a vulnerable position.

I hope you can see by this snippet that body language matters. So do emotions.

Handling Emotions

Some participants will cry. You need to be prepared for this. "Ideally, in qualitative research an interactive conversation is created between participant and interviewer that provides plenty of room for participants to engage in sense making about issues that are important to them," Ellingson (2017: 111) writes. This sense making means that you will be confronted with the emotions surrounding the topic. In other words, you need to know what to do when people cry. Or get angry. Or upset.

Familiarize yourself with nonverbal signals of distress. As an example, shaking one's leg is often a sign of anxiety. Becoming very quiet and closing in on one's self while talking about a difficult topic could be a sign of disassociation. Although we are not therapists, it is ok to acknowledge and validate your participant's pain. You can say things such as "I see this is difficult for you" or "Clearly you are upset." You may feel compelled to give them a hug, but it is best not to touch your participants.

Never leave an interview while someone is in distress, unless you feel you are in danger (e.g., if they are directing their anger toward you). Shift your questions to some that are more neutral to try to calm their emotional response. Offer a break: Maybe they would like to go splash some water on their face or get a drink of water. If you are unable to diffuse the situation, ask the participant if they need to call someone to come get them, or if you can make that call for them. Stay until that person arrives. If that is not an option, make sure you have the number of an emergency crisis line. Call 911 if you need to. Although that level of emotional response is rare, it is important to be prepared.

People may say things you disagree with or that make you feel angry or upset. Withhold your judgment and try to keep your facial expression neutral. If you only want to talk to people who agree with you, you're going to have a skewed view of the issue.

It is not simply the participant's emotions you need to keep an eye on; you must be mindful of your own. Recently, a colleague told me about interviewing a mother whose child had been brutally murdered. The interview lasted four hours, not because it was planned to (my colleague had planned for an hour, maybe an hour and a half) but because the woman wanted someone to hear her. Afterward, my colleague said she felt drained. She cried for a long time, and then she went and did something unrelated to her research to try to feel better.

Practice self-care. We can suffer from vicarious trauma, and sometimes our own past traumas are triggered during our research. Another colleague of mine requires all of her doctoral students working on qualitative dissertations to be in therapy. I don't go that far, but I do want my students to take care of their own emotional needs.

A social worker once told me that you can't cry and take a drink at the same time. I make sure I have something to drink, even if it's just a bottle of water that I've brought with me, so that if I start to get upset on the participant's behalf, I can stop myself from crying. But I have cried with participants. Your own human responses are valid, too.

As much as I emphasized deep listening above, there are times when deep listening is not in your best interest. If you find yourself becoming too upset, stop with the deep listening and think about something unrelated to the project. Think about what you are going to have for dinner, or something else that will completely shift your thoughts. Use whatever works for you. The recorder will still catch their words. This is not meant to be disrespectful; it is meant to protect your own mental health. We want to listen, but we don't want to take on someone else's trauma. Return to deep listening once you feel calm enough to do so.

Your emotions should not overshadow those of your participants. Your participant should never feel responsible for making you feel better. Suck it up and be emotional after they leave.

Another way to practice self-care is to debrief after the interview. Talk with a colleague about what you heard, what went well, what did not. Talk about how you felt about the interview. If you don't have someone you can talk to, journal about the experience. Release the feelings so that you are not carrying them around with you. Remember that although you can have empathy for someone else's pain, it is still *their* pain. You do not have to take that pain on yourself.

How to Become a Better Interviewer

We want to get the best possible interview because this will be our data. The better our data, the better analysis and writing we can do. Thus, it is important that you become a good interviewer. Indeed, the ability to conduct an interview well is one of the most important skills that qualitative researchers need to develop.

At first you may find your interviews are clumsy and awkward. This should improve over time. The key to being a good interviewer is practice. There are some things you can do to improve your interviewing skills:

1. *Listen to expert interviewers.* What do they do well? How do they get the participant talking? Terry Gross, host of the NPR program *Fresh Air*, is well known as one of the best interviewers in media. Often, people she's interviewing will say things such as "No one has ever asked me that before," or they will end the interview with a comment about how much they enjoyed the conversation. You can find her interviews online as podcasts, or listen to her show daily on the radio if you have access.

2. *Practice.* Even with structured interviews, the interview should feel less formal and more conversational. Although you don't want people to forget the interview is for research, you want them to be comfortable enough to talk easily with you. Find people that you can practice interviewing, who can also give you feedback on how you did. I have my students pair up and interview each other, with one taking the role of "participant." After the interview, they have a conversation about what worked well and what didn't.

3. *Listen to the recordings of your interviews.* If you are doing most of the talking, you have a problem. Listen for times you talk over the participant and opportunities you may have missed for further information. Learn from your mistakes.

4. *Don't be afraid of silence.* Use silence to your benefit. We are socialized to keep a conversation going and to fill empty space. But sometimes people need time to think before they answer a question. Don't rush them. Silence may feel uncomfortable to you, but let them be the one to break it.

5. *Find a mentor.* In graduate school, I was a member of a disaster research lab. After a large tornado disaster in Oklahoma, my mentor decided we would do fieldwork and interviews there. Before I was allowed to go off and work on my own, however, she took me with her on a few interviews. This gave me a chance to see how she did them and what she expected me to do. I recommend you do something similar if you are new to interviewing or if you are leading your own team of researchers.

How Many Interviews Are Enough?

Institutional review board applications usually ask how many participants you expect to have in your project. Whereas quantitative researchers can conduct power analysis (a statistical test to determine how many people should be surveyed in order to do the proper analysis), qualitative researchers don't have that luxury. A specific number is difficult to pinpoint. You need as many people as you need to find the answer to your research question.

I am wary of anyone who says there is a set number of participants that qualitative researchers should have. Instead, we are often looking for saturation. This means that we get to a point where adding more people to the study is no longer giving us new information. This can happen at different times—some researchers may find saturation with only a few interviews, whereas others need dozens of interviews. Some research projects will never reach saturation, and the researcher will stop interviewing when they have enough data to write about.

The number of people you interview also depends on the length and depth of the interview. There's a major difference between conducting ten interviews that are fifteen minutes long and conducting ten interviews that are four hours long, conducted over multiple meetings.

So how many interviews should you do? As many as you need to do in order to have a robust answer to your research question.

Focus Groups

Although I do not go into great detail about focus groups in this text, I do want to say a few words about them. A focus group is essentially a group interview. As you proceed through discussion, you hope to find group synergy. In a good focus group, the members will bounce ideas off of each other and off you. It is not unlike a seminar-style class. Olson (2011: 41) writes that "focus groups are conducted when the researcher is interested in the interactions that occur among group members as well as their responses to questions posed by the interviewer." A focus group should not be used as a shorthand to gather a lot of data at once. If you are not interested in group dynamics, you should conduct one-on-one interviews instead.

Typically in focus group studies, the researcher will hold more than one group. As you might imagine, data are more complex than with individual

> A focus group should not be used simply as a way to get a lot of information at once.

interviews. "In addition to the actual text from the interview [the transcripts]," Olson (2011: 42) writes, "the researcher must also consider issues such as the social context of the group, nonverbal data, and the sequential nature of the interactions when developing the interpretation of data."

There are a few issues that you need to additionally be concerned about when conducting focus groups. Just like in a classroom, there can be a problem of one or two people dominating the conversation and silencing others in the group. You can also run into a problem of no one wanting to be the first to talk, or the group simply doesn't coalesce into a flowing conversation. People can easily get off topic, and some may try to have side conversations while the larger conversation is going on. Before going into a focus group setting, be sure you know how you will handle such problems.

When conducting a focus group, most researchers use at least two team members. One member facilitates the group while the second takes notes on what happens. In addition, you should record the session. If it is possible, video the group; video is easier to analyze than audio recordings because of the multiple voices. However, you need to consider whether the group you are working with would be amenable to video recording. Particularly for sensitive topics, group members may not want to be on video. To be safe, you might want to take both types of devices with you and ask the group which they would prefer. If anyone is opposed to video, you should go with audio.

Troubling the Interview

Although interviews are important in qualitative research, they are not without drawbacks. When we conduct interviews, we often expect participants will articulately tell us what they think and why they think the way they do, as if their responses would be unbiased. Whereas researchers are interrogated for bias, the standpoints and biases of participants are seldom addressed. Yet people filter what they tell us (or tell anyone for that matter). Some details stick out while others are forgotten. Over time, the story may change as new meanings are added to the tale. To think that interviews capture The Truth is a fallacy. They capture A truth.

I was once invited by a newspaper to be interviewed for a story it was working on about the COVID-19 pandemic. The request came via email. I wrote the reporter back and said I would be happy to be interviewed; however, I wanted her to send the questions and I would respond to them over email. She emailed me back and argued that it was "industry standard" to do voice interviews without providing the questions ahead of time because she wanted to get my authentic response, and therefore she would not interview me, thank you very much.

There are times when a news reporter or a qualitative researcher would want an immediate response. Reporters often enjoy catching someone off guard. It makes for a better story when someone slips up and says something they perhaps shouldn't have.

This was not that kind of news article, however, and most researchers don't want their participants to make fools of themselves. The reporter wanted me to participate because of my expertise in the field. Indeed, this was a time they should have wanted correct information and not off-the-cuff sound bites.

Be prepared that sometimes interviews will go bad. Some interviews will not give you enough information to be valuable to your study. Maybe you weren't able to gain rapport, or the individual wasn't interested in answering your questions, or you just weren't able to get the information you needed from them. Some people are more articulate than others. It is ok to not use all of your interviews in your analysis. If an interview is not useful, get rid of it and interview someone else. I do not mean to do this if a participant gives you information counter to what you want to hear—that would be a valuable finding. Rather, I mean interviews in which the participant doesn't give you enough information to work with.

Another consideration is how much time has passed since the event you are asking about happened. For example, asking people who have given birth about their birthing experience a few days after the birth will give you different information than asking someone who gave birth five or ten years ago. They will remember in different detail, and over time they will re-create and reinterpret the narrative about the experience.

Skill in interviewing is one of the best tools you can have in your qualitative toolbox. Take the time to learn to conduct interviews well. It will make such a difference in the quality of your data.

References

Arndt, Sonja. 2017. "(Un)becoming Data Through Philosophical Thought Processes of Pasts, Presents and Futures." In *Disrupting Data in Qualitative Inquiry: Entanglements with the Post-Critical and Post-Anthropocentric*, edited by Mirka Koro-Ljungberg, Teija Löytönen, and Marek Tesar, 93–104. New York: Lang.

Ellingson, Laura L. 2017. *Embodiment in Qualitative Research*. New York: Routledge.

Gullion, Jessica Smartt. 2004. School Nurses as Volunteers in a Bioterrorism Event. *Biosecurity and Bioterrorism* 2, no. 2: 112–117.

Le Guin, Ursula K., and David Naimon. 2018. *Conversations on Writing*. Portland, OR: Tin House Books.

Morris, Alan. 2015. *A Practical Introduction to In-Depth Interviewing*. Los Angeles: SAGE.

Olson, Karin. 2011. *Essentials of Qualitative Interviewing*. Walnut Creek, CA: Left Coast Press.

Further Reading

Gross, Terry. 2004. *All I Did Was Ask: Conversations with Writers, Actors, Musicians, and Artists*. New York: Hyperion.

The Paris Review. 2009. *The Paris Review Interviews, Vols. 1–4*. New York: Picador.

Discussion Questions

1. What are the different types of interviews? When is it most appropriate to use them?
2. What are some of the drawbacks to interviewing?

Active Learning

1. Write a research question. Next, compose a questionnaire that would get answers to that question. Practice interviewing your classmates. Revise the questionnaire as needed and practice it again.

Mindfulness Exercises

1. What are your strengths and weaknesses when it comes to interviewing? How could you improve your skills?
2. How comfortable are you with interviewing, particularly with interviewing strangers? What steps could you take to be more comfortable?
3. How does it feel to have someone truly listen to you?

6

Ethnography

Ethnography is often referred to as "deep hanging out." Ethnographers spend a significant amount of time in a community in order to understand their slice of social life. In this chapter, we explore ethnographic practice, fieldwork, participant observation, and conducting ethnography on the internet.

Jeremy and I sit at a picnic table across the street from a gas drilling operation. We are eating snow cones at the small stand that has opened up for the summer. He pauses as an eighteen-wheeled tanker truck turns in to the site, then tells me a story:

"A guy called me one day—I think it was 2007, summer 2007; it can't be that long ago, can it? 2008 maybe—[and] said 'Hey we got notice in our door that someone wants to lease our mineral rights.' This is not too far from my house, and I was like 'well that's crazy, I didn't think that [drilling activity] was over this far [east].'"

He stops talking and takes a few bites of his snow cone. His is blue. Mine is red, strawberry. I hold it against my temple to try to cool off. It is over 102 degrees outside. There is a loud clanging sound, coupled with the sounds of multiple running engines, coming from across the street, and the air is thick with diesel exhaust. Jeremy chose this location for his interview to make a point about just how bad urban drilling is. He's made it.

—Gullion (2015: 109)

This passage is from my 2015 book, *Fracking the Neighborhood: Reluctant Activists and Natural Gas Drilling*. Using ethnography as the research method, I studied the impact of natural gas extraction on the health and well-being of people in the local communities on the Barnett Shale in North Texas. The Barnett Shale is a geological formation with rich deposits of natural gas. Unfortunately for the residents, this was not discovered until after millions of people had built homes and cities on top of the Shale, including the cities of both Dallas and Fort Worth.

Qualitative Research in Health and Illness. Jessica Smartt Gullion, Oxford University Press. © Oxford University Press 2024.
DOI: 10.1093/oso/9780190915988.003.0007

Under Texas law, land is divided into surface rights and mineral rights. Often, the owner of the surface rights does not own the mineral rights. Mineral owners have the legal right to go onto private property and drill for gas (or any other mineral underground that they wish to reach). Thus, the industrial activities associated with natural gas extraction (including fracking) took place in neighborhoods, on school grounds, and in parks—tucked into nooks and crannies of the communities—and threatened the health of the communities.

"Ethnography involves the intentional, systematic collection of information and data on the lived realities of a particular group of people" over a period of time (Gullion 2015: 10). Ethnography allowed me to immerse myself in the phenomenon of living with the industrial activity of fracking in one's neighborhood. Madden (2010: 32) writes that

> being with people (or more precisely, being ethnographic with people), in their time and space, in all their strangeness and in their mundane quotidian flow, is still one of the most valued ways to build a qualitative understanding of the particulars and generalities of the human condition.

Ethnography affords a researcher the chance to live in the setting alongside the participants, to be in the midst of the phenomena they are studying. In this chapter, we explore how to conduct ethnographic research.

As a method, ethnography is used across academic disciplines. Nurse ethnographers, for example, research topics such as nurse practitioners working in acute care settings (Williamson et al. 2012), nursing education (Malinsky, DuBois, and Jacquest 2010), or the role of nurses as social change agents during political revolutions (Pine 2013).

Conducting ethnography is a long-term commitment. You need to have sufficient time to see what unfolds. I spent three years working on my fracking project, with two years in the field and one year spent on analysis and writing the book. Fieldwork involved going to city council meetings and town hall–style meetings held by various state agencies and grassroots organizations, attending (and participating in) protests, and attending meetings with grassroots organizations. I also conducted fieldwork on the internet. This included examining blogs, news reports (and the comments), government organizations' websites, grassroots organizations' websites, and industry websites. I collected an inordinate number of reports—every report and white paper I could find—including those produced by oil and gas companies. To supplement the fieldwork, I conducted twenty in-depth interviews (lasting one to three hours each) with people I had identified as "key players" in the natural gas extraction debates. These people were highly visible, often spoke at meetings and events, and most maintained blogs. I also interviewed members of some of the regulatory agencies to get their perspectives. I transcribed all of the interviews. Many of the public meetings were transcribed by the host agency and archived on their websites, so I used those as data. I had informal conversations with people as well. I visited active drilling sites and fracking operations and also gas wells that had been completed (with completed wells the drills are gone and a pump, often run on

Ethnography is a long-term commitment.

diesel fuel, is put in place to move the gas into transport pipelines). Often, an activist would accompany me on these visits and explain the history of the site. I collected handouts and fliers at events. I kept extensive field notes (several notebooks full) and interpersonal reflection notes. These included observations, maps I'd drawn of relationships, random thoughts, occasional drawings, and theoretical ideas. I would also jot down information from informal conversations, without identifying who I spoke with. I included notes to myself to follow up on things people told me about. I took hundreds of photographs.

While I kept field notes by hand, I wrote theoretical memos on the computer. In memoing, the researcher writes out theoretical ideas about what is happening in the field, about the interconnections they are seeing, and how the data they've gathered so far hang together. These memos eventually morphed into the book. I read as much scientific literature on gas extraction and activism as I could. I have Bankers Boxes filled with data from this project (identifiable data have since been shredded and disposed of). The sheer volume of data (literally thousands of pages) was at times overwhelming and required a good data management plan (we talk more about how to do that later).

As you can see from the example above, conducting an ethnography can be an enormous project. But it is also the richest way to conduct research. If you have a research question that lends itself to ethnographic research, you are in for a wonderful experience.

Why Ethnography?

Van Maanen (2011: 2) argues "fieldwork is one answer—some say the best—to the question of how the understanding of others, close or distant, is achieved." This is because the researcher immerses themself in a specific setting over a period of time to understand a phenomena or culture of interest. The goal of ethnography is to discover what it is like to be part of the group that you are studying and to tell the story of that group. As a research method, ethnography involves being with people in their place (wherever or whatever that place may be). Hanging out. Watching. Perhaps participating. Talking to people. Trying to understand one slice of social life.

The field is the physical or virtual space in which the research takes place. For example, in Mol's (2003) ethnography of the ontology of arteriosclerosis, the field was a Dutch university hospital. This is where she spent time observing, asking questions, and collecting data. The field for my fracking project is called multisited. It took place in different cities and online.

Living is a dynamic process; life changes moment to moment. If you interview me today, I may be in a good mood, which in turn has an impact on how I respond to your interview questions. Tomorrow, I may be having a bad day, which could have a different impact on my responses. With fieldwork, a researcher can document those dynamics changes over time. You get to know people and their moods. You learn how events unfold. The ethnographer witnesses, uncovers, and seeks to understand the motion and fluidity of life.

> The ethnographer witnesses, uncovers, and documents the motion and fluidity of life.

"Ethno" means people or culture. "Graphy" means to write about. A substantial component of this method is writing, and writing as a way of knowing. We are keepers of stories (Gullion 2015). Madden (2010: 153) writes,

> The act of writing is more than simply reporting on the interpretations that spring from the primary and secondary ethnographic data. The act of ethnographic writing is a form of collating, reporting, and interpreting at the same time; it is both systematic and artful.

We can think of ethnography as embodied storytelling, as well as embodied theorizing. Indeed, "the more theoretically relevant a piece of ethnographic work is, the more it is able to travel from local community concerns and substantive areas to capture wider academic interest and make a more lasting contribution to scholarship," Puddephatt, Shaffir, and Kleinknecht (2009: 2) remind us. Because we are academics and not journalists, we also situate our work in larger academic conversations.

Gullion (2022: 18) writes,

> Ethnography occupies an interesting interrogative space at the intersection of the sciences, humanities, and the arts. Because of the lived reality of the groups and activities we research, and their dynamic nature, good ethnographers utilize all three domains in their research. We can (and good ethnographers do) also use tools from all three domains. Sometimes the answers we seek aren't where we look. Embracing interdisciplinarity and even transcending disciplinary boundaries leads to both a richer ethnography and also to a richer understanding of our research subject.

A Very Brief History of Ethnography

Ethnography is rooted in the fields of anthropology and sociology. Historically, anthropologists used ethnography to study preliterate cultures, whereas sociologists studied urban subcultures (typically subaltern). This is no longer the case; ethnography is used to study all sorts of cultures and phenomena.

I'm going to keep this history section brief because there are many texts that chronicle it in depth. This is a general overview and not meant to be comprehensive. However, the main points I wish to get across are the following:

1. Ethnography is one of the oldest social science research methods.
2. The history of ethnography is rife with othering and colonization.
3. Ethnographers today are diverse, and they push back against that colonialist history.

We begin with a look at anthropology. The first ethnographies, if they could be called such, were travelogs. People would travel to some "exotic" locale and write about what they'd witnessed. As anthropology emerged as an academic discipline, ethnography became more systematized and scientific. Travel to a distant land to explore an unknown culture was a rite of passage for budding anthropologists (Van Maanen 2011). They believed that by understanding "primitive" cultures, they could determine how "civilized" cultures evolved.

Although there is some debate about who founded the field, Bronislaw Malinowski's book, *Argonauts of the Western Pacific* (1922/2016), has been touted as one of the first examples of in-depth, scientific field research. "By the late 1920s fieldwork and the image of the scientifically trained fieldworker stalking the wiley native in his natural habitat had become the cornerstone of anthropology," Van Maanen (2011: 17) writes. To this day, it is the norm in many anthropology departments that one builds a research agenda doing fieldwork in a remote area of the world.

In contrast, early sociologists turned their ethnographic gaze on subcultures (typically deviant subcultures) in their own neighborhoods. In the United States, a group of researchers known as the Chicago School (from the University of Chicago) engaged in urban ethnography. Park, Thomas, Burgess, and their students considered the city an intriguing, exotic setting worthy of exploration (Van Maanen 2011). They wrote in a documentary, journalistic style and sought to uncover "social facts," following Durkheim's tome, *The Rules of Sociological Method* (1895/1982).

Power in early ethnographic research was asymmetrical; the ethnographer was the observer of the "others." Both disciplines have imperialistic roots, and a large body of critical research has since addressed this. Today's ethnographers seek to minimize violence on research participants, and they often work in collaboration with the participants. This often involves co-constructed narratives, member checking, community-based action research, and other built-in assurances that the relationship is beneficial to both researchers and participants.

As the two disciplines evolved, ethnography took hold as the gold standard for research in anthropology. While some sociologists still engaged in ethnographic research, many sociologists embraced positivism and turned to quantitative methods through survey research. Meanwhile, ethnography as method has transcended disciplinary boundaries and has become a useful tool for researchers across the university. Some ethnographers turn inward, researching their own communities, or even using their own lives as data—such as with autoethnography. We more closely examine autoethnography in Chapter 8.

Ethnographers immerse themselves in a social group that they may or may not have had prior relations with, and they attempt to achieve an understanding of what it is like to be part of that group. They then interpret and translate that experience through writing and other forms of representation for others. By conducting this work over time, ethnographers participate in the foldings and unfoldings of the processes within and around the group. Life is dynamic, variable, and changing, and ethnographers attempt to understand that movement through engaged practice (Gullion 2015, 2018).

Often, students think they are doing ethnography because they've read a lot of information and conducted interviews. Although that is fantastic work, that is not ethnography. When researchers are engaged in ethnography, they are *living the story* with the participants (Butler-Kisber 2010: 78). They engage in meaningful interactions in a particular field or fields for a sustained period of time. It's "often about making the familiar strange and coming to know, through sustained engagement, the who, the where and how of ordinary everyday human interactions, societies, and cultures," Renold and Mellor (2013: 36) write.

Doing Ethnography

Now that we have a basic understanding of the goals of ethnography, let's look at how one can conduct an ethnographic study.

Identifying the Field

The field is the physical or virtual location in which you conduct your research. You can have multiple fields (this is called a multisited ethnography), and your field can be an on-line space.

Once you have identified what it is you would like to research, you need to define the parameters of your field. Perhaps you will work at a particular hospital or in a specific jail health center. Maybe you will hang out with intravenous drug users in a shooting gallery or live for a while in a refugee camp. Your field could be an online message board for people with a particular illness or condition.

The field is an important aspect of the research. It influences what happens to the people within it. Not only will you get to know the people but also you will learn how the place shapes what happens there.

Entering the Field

Once you have identified the field, you need to enter it. How you do this will be shaped by the nature of the field itself.

Let's suppose you are conducting an ethnographic study of Sexual Assault Nurse Examiners (SANE nurses) in a particular emergency room. You are interested in how they interact with the patient victim, the other health care providers, rape crisis counselors, and law enforcement. In this scenario, we assume that your institution's institutional review board (IRB) has already approved the study and you have protocols in place for patient privacy.

The first thing you need to do is get buy-in from the hospital that it is ok for you to do your study there. To get that buy-in, you will probably have to meet with the top administrator, explain exactly what you will be doing, and get their permission. Your IRB might ask for that approval in writing, in which case the administrator should write a letter indicating that they understand what you plan to do and that they are supportive of your work. You should also set up a meeting with the emergency room director and the nursing supervisor. Although they can't stop you from conducting your research once you have the ok from the hospital, they can make life difficult for you if they don't want you there. Talk with them about ways you can do your work both respectfully and without getting in anyone's way. Schedule when you will begin.

On your first day, rather than worry about what the SANE nurses are doing, introduce yourself to them. Explain what you are doing and why you are doing it. Introduce yourself to every employee you meet. Let them know you are conducting research, and get informed consent if your IRB requires it (often the IRB will not require it for informal conversations and observations, but given the setting, it may, so be sure you have approval before entering the field).

It is useful to find a gatekeeper who can help you gain entrance to the field. A gatekeeper is someone already present in the field who knows people and can introduce you and vouch for you. This can be extremely valuable. For the SANE study, if you knew a SANE nurse working at that hospital before you began, they could advocate to leadership that this is a valuable project, and they can help you get acclimated to the setting. There is one caveat to using a gatekeeper: If they are not well-liked, your relationship with them can harm your study because others view you as an ally to that person. Likewise, it is a problem if the gatekeeper you identify is the wrong person—they represent themselves as a gatekeeper but in fact have no influence in this setting. Or if the gatekeeper does not want you there, they might inhibit your access to places and others.

Remember that ethnography takes place over an extended period of time. At first, you will spend most of your time observing and asking questions for clarification. You want to get the lay of the land, so to speak, before you start interviewing or theorizing. Spend time building rapport. Get to know the people you will be working with. Join them when they go for coffee or a meal (ask if it's ok). Become one of them while still maintaining your identity as a researcher.

Keep extensive field notes. It is difficult to know in the beginning what to write down, but over time you will find yourself focusing on particular aspects of the phenomenon you are studying. We'll explore field notes in more detail below.

Leaving the Field

At some point, you will decide you have enough information and will leave the field. Because life keeps going whether you are there or not, define a concrete end date to your fieldwork. If you don't, you could be in the field forever, and you still need to write up your findings.

After spending so much time in a place, you've probably formed friendships. It's ok to continue those relationships. Just be sure that when you are done collecting data, you are done; don't take advantage of those relationships once you've left the field.

When You Are a Member of the Group You Are Studying

Being a pre-existing member of the group you are studying has its advantages and disadvantages. The advantages include the fact that you already have access to the group. You also have insider knowledge that can make the group easier to navigate. A disadvantage is that you may have on blinders, and because of your insider status, you may not see some of the group dynamics. If this is the case, you might consider using a team of researchers. Or you could mitigate this by using member checks—asking the people participating in the research whether or not they think your observations are accurate.

While conducting my fracking ethnography, I vacillated between being a member of the group and being an outsider. There is a natural geologic edge to the shale at a lake. My house is on the non-shale side of the lake. There are no natural gas deposits under my home or neighborhood. Every day, I cross a bridge over that lake to go to my university, which is on the shale (at one time there was an active well on campus—it is now shut down). Prior to high school, both of my children also crossed that bridge daily to go to school. Most of our daily living activities—grocery shopping, going out to restaurants and other entertainment, visiting friends, etc.—happened on the shale side of the bridge.

During the time I was conducting the study, fracking was at the forefront of both local and national news. It came up in casual conversation. At one meeting, I found out that a well was to be fracked within a couple of blocks of my children's school. At that moment, I flipped from researcher to concerned parent. I acknowledge this in my book so that readers can understand my positionality relative to the topic.

How the Field Shapes the Work

Consider the place and space and how interactions change or are changed by the space in which they occur. For example, Ellingson (2017) writes about how differently one might interpret the act of a mother holding her crying infant in her home compared to a physician holding a crying infant in an emergency room. The place and the actants within that space influence what a researcher sees.

One thing I found during my research on fracking was that people had to learn where decisions were made and how to access the spaces that decision-makers inhabited. One participant told me she had to figure out where city hall was located—she had never had reason to go there. Meetings may be held at times of the day when most people work, which structurally limits their participation. City council and other governing bodies have rules about who can speak and when. It took time for the activists to learn how to work with the governing bodies.

As we move into the field, we also need to think about how much we are going to participate in events. I remained an observer as much as possible; however, there were times at protests where someone would give me a sign and I would participate. I was asked to help develop policy, but I declined because I felt that put me too much in the action.

Participation can raise all sorts of situational ethics dilemmas for you. For example, if you are studying drug culture, will you try the drugs? Although it may be illegal, it would get you credibility with the group. You would understand how the drug feels and thus have a better understanding of why people use it (note that I am not advocating that you do this; I'm just bringing it up as an example). What about other behaviors? If you are investigating tattoo culture, will you get a tattoo? If you are investigating injuries to boxers, will you get in the ring? Participation can help the researcher have an embodied feel for what it is like to do what the participants are doing.

Data

Ethnographers hoard data. And anything related to your project could be data. Let's go back to our SANE example and look at what all could be collected and analyzed.

Ask for a tour of the space. You might be able to get a map of the hospital; if not, draw one. You could then draw the paths the nurses take on it. You could do the same with doctors, emergency medical services personnel, and the patients. How do people move through the hospital? Record all this in your field notes.

You could take photographs of the spaces (obviously not of the patients). Take photos of the exam room, the rape kit, the gowns victims are given, and anything else that catches your eye. If there are pamphlets or other handouts, get copies of them.

Talk to people. Conduct in-depth interviews of the SANE nurses, but also have informal conversations with them. Record and transcribe the in-depth interviews; write about the informal conversations in your field notes. Talk to the people around the nurses—the doctors, emergency medical services personnel, the police. Take field notes on what they tell you.

Read everything you can find about SANE nursing. See if you can get copies of training manuals. Join the national organization. Find out what others have written about this topic. Discover if there is anything contentious about this type of work. Learn all you can about the subject.

Field Notes

I tend to have a notebook with me at all times in the field. I have smaller sized notebooks that fit in my purse. If I'm in a meeting or some other place where writing in a notebook isn't conspicuous, I will do so; however, most of the time I will write when I have a moment alone. I have balanced a notebook in my lap in restrooms and done a lot of writing in my car. Whereas I prefer to handwrite my notes, some people will work on their laptops or tablets, take notes on their phones, or make voice memos that can be transcribed later.

One of the most difficult parts of beginning an ethnography is figuring out what you should write down. What should you take note of? That's always a challenge in the beginning of an ethnography because you don't know yet what will be important and what won't be. It's normal to feel a little overwhelmed in the beginning. You will probably gather a lot of information that you won't end up using in your final report; that's alright. I typically start off broadly and narrow my focus as my overall picture of the events begins to take shape.

Some items to note include the following:

1. Location
   a. What is the physical space like?
   b. How accessible is the space?
   c. Are you inside or outdoors?
      i. If you are outside, what is the weather like?
   d. Draw a map.
   e. What does it feel like to be in and to move through that space?
2. Participants
   a. Who is there?
   b. How many people are there?
   c. What are their roles?
   d. What do they look like?
   e. How do they arrange themselves?

3. Action
   a. What are people doing?
   b. How do they interact with each other?
   c. How do they interact with objects or other beings (e.g., animals)?
   d. How do they interact with the environment?

This is by no means a complete list of notes you should gather; rather, it is a starting point.

Public Spaces and Private Spaces

An ethical issue specific to ethnographers has to do with researching in public. For example, suppose you are interested in studying how injuries are handled during football games. Part of your observations would take place in the stands, recording how the audience responds when a player gets hurt. Do you tell all those people you are a researcher?

One way to handle this is to ask that an announcement be made during the game that there is a researcher present. If there is a printed program, you could find out if you could put a notice in it. But you don't usually have to do either; ask yourself if the people in that space would have a reasonable expectation of privacy. In this case, the answer is no. You could record how the audience responds; however, if you eavesdrop on someone's private conversation, they must be able to give informed consent if you are going to record that conversation and use it in your research. Private conversations take place in public spaces, so be clear about what you are there to observe.

One general rule I use for myself is to look for the presence of the media. If journalists are there, there should be no expectation of privacy. There are usually journalists at meetings held by government agencies (e.g., city council meetings). I also try to determine whether or not the event or a transcript of the event will be posted online where anyone could access it. If it's publicly available, you can use it without having to get consent.

This is different from spaces that are considered private or where entry is controlled. If you were to go down to the field to hang out with the medical staff during a football game, they need to know what you are there for and give permission for you to be there. The football players should know who you are and what you are doing too. They should all have the opportunity to give informed consent—or to state that they do not want to be part of your research. When in doubt about whether or not informed consent is needed, consult your IRB.

Covert fieldwork, masking that you are there to do research or pretending to be someone you are not, is unethical. And frankly, a good researcher should not need to conduct covert research.

Conducting Ethnographic Research on the Internet

Increasingly, researchers look to the internet as a space to gather data. Some of these data are pre-existing, and other data are gathered through interaction with people online. The internet can also be a great place to recruit potential participants.

Businesses have harnessed the power of big data (sometimes with notable security breaches and invasions of privacy) in order to market products, predict voting patterns, and otherwise attempt subtle (or not so subtle) manipulation of users. This is one way that information on social media becomes skewed. Algorithms provide the user with the same "type" of information and products based on user activity in a feedback loop. Much content is now tailored to the individual based on their activity on the internet. Be aware of this if you are conducting research on the internet. The results you get in searches or in your social media feeds could be quite different from what others see.

Netnography is a type of ethnographic research conducted on the internet. Kozinets (2020: 133–134) identifies four elements of netnography:

1. Cultural focus
2. Social media data
3. Immersive engagement
4. Netnography praxis

Kozinets identifies six different components for researchers to explore (pp. 133–134):

a. The use of new language and symbols, such as novel words, acronyms, memes, fonts, or emojis, which may be created exclusively for online use, or reflected online, or

b. The expression of online rituals, such as posting particular types of video, image or avatar; some of these will be practices that are only possible online, or are enabled by various facets of online experience such as anonymity or partial anonymity, or

c. The adoption of new identities, expressed through role modeling and play acting, adopting new fashions, attempting new social positions (such as an influencer, or an activists), sometimes through aggression, and often in a dynamic manner, as if trying on new identities were a stylistic matter, or

d. The telling of stories, sharing of beliefs, passing along of powerful images and media; social media is filled with narratives whose importance requires deep analysis, identification and (re)connection of meaning; and

e. The inculcations and reinforcement of value and value systems through the feedback reward structures of social media sharing, commenting, and liking; which is also tied into

f. Relations of power, group dynamics, exclusion and inclusion, submission and domination, and hierarchies that express themselves online.

There may be other things that you find that haven't been identified here.

When thinking about ethical research on the internet, the first consideration is whether or not the site is public. Just as there is a distinction between public and private spaces in other fieldwork, the same applies to conducting ethnography on the internet. Has the information you are interested in been shared on a public platform, without any password protection? If it is publicly available, where anyone could access it without going through passwords or firewalls, you can use the data without obtaining informed consent.

If the site is private, or if there is an expectation of privacy (even if the site is not truly private), then people need to have a chance to give informed consent for their information to be used in research. They have rights as research participants. Does the site have a moderator? If so, you may need their permission to reach out to the rest of the group members. Do not skip this step; you may find yourself banned from the group.

One of my guilty pleasures is playing *World of Warcraft*, an MMORPG (massively multiplayer online role-playing game). This means that many (millions) of people play the game simultaneously, and a player can interact in a number of different ways with other players. It would be a fascinating field to conduct research, and indeed many people have. In addition to the ability to interact with random people, you can specifically interact with real-life friends in the space as well. Often, friends and I will "meet" there and help each other through the game and/or chat about all sorts of different topics while we are online. For example, in the summer of 2020, there was a lot of discussion about how our local governments and schools were handling COVID-19 and about the Black Lives Matters protests that were happening in our cities.

There are a variety of ways to communicate in the game. There is a chat window, where people can type to each other. This can be "whispered" to only one player, broadcast to anyone nearby or in the same zone you are in, or posted to a specified group or guild. In addition, many players use systems such as Discord that allow for voice communication (and in some cases, video). Players often wear headsets designed for this purpose. Like the chat box, Discord has different levels of communication, with varying levels of privacy.

I mentioned guilds—most players are members of a guild. My guild has approximately thirty core members. We talk in-game through the chat box and live in a private Discord channel. We use these to play the game (sometimes while going through a "raid" or other quest together), and we talk about all sorts of other things, from gaming to who just had a baby. Some of the guild members have met face-to-face (we have an annual in-person guild party, where people come from all over the United States and Canada). Some have never met in person but talk daily, and they have done so for years.

World of Warcraft could be an ethnographic field. There are many other spaces like this online. A researcher would need to get consent from the other players to be part of the research, and they would have to protect the other players' privacy. Guilds are private. A player has to be invited into a guild. There are rules for membership and behavior, and players who violate those rules are kicked out. Therefore, you need to get permission to do research there.

This is where understanding a group's culture and norms is important. Suppose I wanted to conduct research on communication and hierarchy in my guild. I would begin by reaching out to the "guild master" (the person who created and thus "owns" the guild) and tell them my idea. The guild master would be my gatekeeper and would run the idea past the officers (we have five). If they decided the project was a good idea, I could inform everyone in the guild that I wanted to conduct research with them. One way I could do this is by using a "pinned" message that everyone would see when they first log in.

Next, I would need to review consent and get signed forms from everyone. I could do this while we were all in Discord, email them the form and ask them to email it back, or use a software program that allows users to sign electronically. I would need to figure out what to do about members who chose not to participate but who are still interacting with the others. That alone might kill my study. As you can see, this has the potential to be both a fascinating study and a massive headache.

Although it might be tempting, it would be unethical for me to conduct research on my guild covertly. Confidentiality, beneficence, nonmalfeasance, informed consent, integrity—all of the ethical precepts we've discussed apply in an online environment. Where things get tricky is the delineation of public versus private space. Normally, an ethnographer (just like a journalist) can make observations in a public space without getting informed consent from everyone present. In a public space where anyone can attend, there is (usually) no expectation of privacy. It is when we attempt to enter private (or presumed private) spaces that we must avoid conducting covert research.

Another consideration is the sensitivity of the topic. Thinking back to my guild example above, behavior during a raid is less sensitive than discussing someone's depression in the group. Although we can (and should) conduct research on sensitive topics, we need to ensure that the participants know what we are doing, have consented to it, and are protected from harm.

A tricky consideration when conducting research on the internet is whether or not we are working with vulnerable populations. Due to the anonymity possible on the internet, you may have vulnerable people in your study without knowing it. It is easy to hide one's identity and age on the internet.

Like any other research, when we conduct research on the internet, we must weigh the risks of the study relative to the benefits. In many cases, the risks will be minimal; however, we still must take them into account and let our IRB decide if our mitigation strategies are appropriate. Likewise, we must also protect people's privacy.

There are some places on the internet that can easily be considered public spaces. My local newspaper, for example, has an online presence. Newspapers are intended for public consumption and are not private. My hometown newspaper also has a feature that enables anyone to post comments on articles. Are those comments also public, and thus not protected by privacy rules? Most IRBs would say yes, they are in the public domain and the people who posted the comments should have no expectation for privacy. If it is public, then it is fair game for researchers.

Public versus private space is the crux of human subjects protections on the internet. My personal opinion on the matter is that if there is any expectation of privacy (e.g., having to use a password to access the space or only allowing approved "friends" or members to access the space), then the data should be treated as private and allowed all of the protections we afford any other private information. If you wish to use this type of data, your study must be reviewed by an IRB, and you must have informed consent from all of the participants.

Kozinets (2020: 164) writes that "online fieldwork is an opportunity to be a goodwill ambassador or an ignorant exploiter." Just because you can access someone's information does not mean that you should use it for research purposes. Let people know you are a researcher and get informed consent from them to use their information.

"Data scraping" is a technique in which a researcher uses specialized software or manually collects large amounts of data, such as all of the comments on a video or post, or all of the tweets with a particular hashtag. Those data are then analyzed for trends. This is another way researchers work on the internet.

To be sure, there have been many data breaches and (what some would say are) nefarious uses of people's online data. The Cambridge Analytica/Facebook scandal is one example. Cambridge Analytica used Facebook data to create voter profiles in order to help the Trump presidential campaign. Many people were incensed to learn that what they considered to be private data were used in such a manner.

Some would argue that nothing on the internet is truly private. However, there are spaces that people think of as secure. Certainly, online medical records, telemedicine, and telepharmacy are examples of data with strong encryption designed to protect people's privacy. And people trust such data will be kept private. But aside from that, most people's day-to-day online activities are not as secure, and indeed are often public.

We also cannot rely on usernames to protect privacy. Often, people's usernames are not their real names. Although one might think that would afford privacy, usernames could be identifiable in that community. Returning to my *World of Warcraft* example, all of my characters have names. My guild knows my real name, but people outside my guild would not have that information unless I gave it to them. However, other people know me in-game as my characters' names, and using those names in a write-up of research could potentially affect my online relationships and reputation in the game.

The following are additional questions to ask yourself when conducting online research:

1. Are you collecting IP addresses? IP addresses are often linked to content, can be captured without the user's knowledge, and can be used to identify the user. Users should be able to give informed consent for you to collect this information.
2. Are you certain you are dealing with adults? What about protected populations on the internet? Children and other protected populations must still be protected online. In addition, children younger than age thirteen years in the United States have extra protections under the Children's Online Privacy Protection Rule, along with other legislation.
3. When interacting with participants online, they should have the same protections as if the research were being conducted in any other setting. How will you get their informed consent?
4. It is possible that what you are analyzing didn't come from human users at all but, rather, was generated by bots. During the COVID-19 pandemic, for example, bot-generated memes told people about the dangers of masks—the opposite of what public health officials advised. Some people believed these memes were true. Know that you may be interacting with a bot.

In addition to collecting data from the internet, many researchers use it as a tool for conducting interviews and focus groups.

In March 2020, my university's IRB, like many others throughout the country, suspended face-to-face interviewing because of the risk of COVID-19. In order to keep their research projects going, many researchers turned to online interviews, using programs such as Zoom to conduct their interviews. Protocols that had already been approved for face-to-face interviewing were changed to reflect this new medium. In many cases, the interviewers would email the consent form to the participant prior to the interview and ask the participant to sign it electronically and email it back before the interview. The start of the interview would involve reviewing the consent form and allowing the participant a chance to ask questions about the research before the interview continued. The interview could be recorded for later analysis. Programs such as Zoom could also be used to create transcriptions of the recordings.

Ethnography is data- and time-intensive research. But it also provides a depth and richness that other techniques cannot. If you want to understand a particular slice of social life, this is a great way to do it.

References

Butler-Kisber, Lynn. 2010. *Qualitative Inquiry: Thematic, Narrative and Arts-Informed Perspectives*. Los Angeles: SAGE.

Durkheim, Emile. 1895/1982. *The Rules of Sociological Method*, translated by W. D. Halls. New York: Free Press.

Ellingson, Laura L. 2017. *Embodiment in Qualitative Research*. New York: Routledge.

Gullion, Jessica Smartt. 2015. *Fracking the Neighborhood: Reluctant Activists and Natural Gas Drilling*. Cambridge, MA: MIT Press.

Gullion, Jessica Smartt. 2018. *Diffractive Ethnography: Social Sciences in the Ontological Turn*. London: Routledge.

Gullion, Jessica. 2022. *Writing Ethnography*, 2nd ed. Leiden, the Netherlands: Brill.

Kozinets, Robert V. 2020. *Netnography: The Essential Guide to Qualitative Social Media Research*, 3rd ed. Los Angeles: SAGE.

Madden, Raymond. 2010. *Being Ethnographic: A Guide to the Theory and Practice of Ethnography*. Los Angeles: SAGE.

Malinowski, Bronislaw. 1922/2016. *Argonauts of the Western Pacific: An Account of Native Enterprise and Adventure in the Archipelagos of Melanesia New Guinea*. London: Oxford University Press.

Malinsky, Lynn, Ruth DuBois, and Diane Jacquest. 2010. "Building Scholarship Capacity and Transforming the Nurse Educator's Practice Through Institutional Ethnography." *International Journal of Nursing Education Scholarship* 7, no. 1: 1–12.

Mol, Annemarie. 2003. *The Body Multiple: Ontology in Medical Practice*. Durham, NC: Duke University Press.

Pine, A. 2013. "Revolution as a Care Plan: Ethnography, Nursing, and Somatic Solidarity in Honduras." *Social Science and Medicine* 99: 143–152.

Puddephatt, Antony J., William Shaffir, and Steven W. Kleinknecht. 2009. *Ethnographies Revisited: Constructing Theory in the Field*. London: Routledge.

Renold, Emma, and David Mellor. 2013. "Deleuze and Guattari in the Nursery: Towards a Multi-Sensory Mapping of Young Gendered and Sexual Becomings." In *Deleuze and Research Methodologies*, edited by Rebecca Coleman and Jessica Ringrose, 23–40. Edinburgh, UK: Edinburgh University Press.

Van Maanen, John. 2011. *Tales of the Field: On Writing Ethnography*, 2nd ed. Chicago: University of Chicago Press.

Williamson, Susan, Timothy Twelvetree, Jacqueline Thompson, and Kinta Beaver. 2012. "An Ethnographic Study Exploring the Role of Ward-Based Advanced Nurse Practitioners in an Acute Medical Setting." *Journal of Advanced Nurse Practitioners* 68, no. 7: 1579–1588.

FURTHER READING

Desmond, Matthew. 2016. *Evicted: Poverty and Profit in the American City*. New York: Broadway Books.

Dunier, Mitchell. 1999. *Sidewalk*. New York: Farrar, Straus & Giroux.

Goffman, Alice. 2014. *On the Run: Fugitive Life in an American City*. New York: Picador.

Discussion Questions

1. What are the steps in an ethnography?
2. How would you go about conducting ethnographic research online?

Active Learning

1. Read an ethnographic study (*hint*: there are some good ones in the Further Reading section). Write about the author's methodology. How transparent was the author about how they conducted their research?
2. Go to a public place and observe for thirty minutes. Take field notes. This can be done with a partner. Do not talk during the exercise. Compare field notes when you are done. How are they similar? Different?

Mindfulness Exercises

1. How might you use ethnography to study something you are interested in?
2. How could you mitigate against colonialism in your own ethnographic practice?

7

Community-Based Action Research

> In this chapter, we explore community-based action research, a collaborative method in which a researcher assists with a community-led project. This often involves a social justice component. We discuss why a researcher might choose this method and how to go about doing it. We also examine common pitfalls in community work and how to move past them.

Community-based action research (also known as action research, participatory action research, or community research) is one way that researchers and community members can collaborate on research projects and engage in community change activities. Gullion and Tilton (2020: 11) write that this "involves situating research within a geographically bounded community to investigate an issue or problem, develop interventions, and assess outcomes." Community-based action research is particularly helpful for both identifying community-wide health concerns and addressing them.

Community-based action research involves co-constructed knowledge building. Community members work alongside academic researchers in a nonhierarchical relationship. Together they decide on the parameters of the problem and how to best investigate it. They then devise an intervention—the action piece of community-based action research—and implement it in their community. This type of research is local and relevant to a particular community. Although researchers may uncover information that could be valuable for other communities, this type of work is not meant to be generalizable to other populations.

Community-based action research has been used to address a wide variety of community problems, including public health issues ranging from homelessness (Moxley and Washington 2013) to the impacts of violence in communities (Mardiros 2001) and child sexual abuse (Reid, Reddock, and Nickenig 2014).

Qualitative Research in Health and Illness. Jessica Smartt Gullion, Oxford University Press. © Oxford University Press 2024.
DOI: 10.1093/oso/9780190915988.003.0008

Many methods can be employed in this type of research, but the hallmark of community-based action research is that the researcher does not design and carry out the research alone. Rather, community members are brought together and decide what information would be valuable to their cause and how to collect it. In this case, the researcher can share their knowledge about different ways to collect the information the community needs. For example, the group might decide that photovoice would be a good technique for capturing people's experiences. The researcher could teach the community members how to use this method, and then the community members would go collect the data. In this way, there is an exchange between the researcher and the community members. The researcher teaches them a skill that they can use in the future. This differs from extractive research projects, in which a researcher enters a community, collects knowledge, and then leaves.

When conceptualizing community-based action research, the primary concern is that the project is collaborative and nonhierarchical. The researcher is a member of a team, not the lead. "This fundamentally alters the power dynamic in research from a 'power over' to 'power with' dynamic, and changes the way in which we understand the entire research process—as collaborative rather than directive, as culturally produced rather than universal," Gullion and Tilton (2020: 20) write.

I mentioned previously in this book that I used to be an epidemiologist at a local health department. Working in public health, I saw health outreach programs fail much too often. That failure was a direct result of not engaging with the community at the outset. Instead, experts (who usually did not live in the community) would create health interventions without input from the community members with whom they wanted to intervene and then be surprised when those interventions didn't work. Often, an intervention works well in one community, so it is "boxed up" (sometimes literally, many of the tools come in a box with a handle) and made available (often sold) to other communities. The problem is that every community is unique and what works well in one community may be a dismal failure in another.

One of the programs that I oversaw at the health department was HIV Outreach and Prevention. The goal of that program was to implement educational programs to halt the spread of HIV and to test people for HIV so that those who were infected could get treatment. The program was funded by the state health department.

When that program was established, researchers with the state health department divided the state into service regions. My community was included in the Dallas, Texas, area service region. Using statistical data, the state experts determined that the primary mode of HIV transmission in this service region was among Black intravenous (IV) drug users. As such, funding for our HIV program stipulated that we were to reach out to this group and perform an educational program tailored to this group. The program materials were literally in a box with a handle so the health educator could take it with them. It included scripts and videos. The program had been demonstrated to reduce HIV transmission in other communities.

There are all sorts of evidence-based community health intervention programs available for use. These have been predeveloped and tested, and they often contain toolkits that can be tailored to one's own community. They are called evidence-based because they have been tested and shown to work. Many are available for free; others can come with a hefty charge. You can find a comprehensive list of evidence-based community health interventions on the National Institutes of Health website.[1]

I do not wish to imply that these programs are bad; in fact, there are some wonderful interventions out there. Should you decide to use one of them, you should make sure that it is appropriate for your community. The trouble with these sorts of programs is that communities are not homogeneous. What works well in one area might fail in another. This doesn't mean it was a bad program; it just wasn't right for that community. It is important to understand the dynamics in your community before using one of these toolkits, no matter how good the intervention sounds.

When we use taxpayer dollars to fund health interventions in the community and those programs fail, it is right for the public to be concerned. When this happens, it is not surprising that some would bring accusations of inappropriate use of funds or say that social programs broadly do not work or that "big government" is a problem.

In the case of our HIV program, the experts had not drilled down into the data enough. To be sure, in Dallas, the primary main source of HIV transmission was among Black IV drug users. But Dallas' greater numbers erased the fact that in our nearby community at that time, HIV transmission was primarily occurring among Hispanic men who have sex with men but who identified as heterosexual.

The experts weren't wrong about the overall trends in the large geographic area they'd chosen, but their recommendations were not appropriate for our smaller geographic area. In terms of the demographics, at that time the percentage of African Americans in our service area was low. And the drug of choice was methamphetamine, not heroin.

HIV outreach and prevention activities look different for IV drug users compared to men who have sex with men. But the state specified that we were to target our program to Black IV drug users—that we work with local law enforcement to identify hot spots of drug activity and teach IV drug users how to clean their works (their drug paraphernalia). Meanwhile, what we really needed to do to bring down transmission rates in our jurisdiction was target safe sex for the Hispanic population. We needed to be in bars and truck stops handing out condoms and performing rapid HIV screening, but the state wouldn't fund that.

The program failed. We did not reach our target numbers of Black IV drug users (the employees used to complain that there were so few in our jurisdiction that they'd already talked to all of them). Meanwhile, HIV rates increased in Hispanic men who had sex with men. The program was eventually disbanded, and the health department no longer had any type of community HIV outreach.

Examples such as this one lead to the criticism of misspending of taxpayer money. It is difficult to disagree with that. This is another reason why it is imperative to understand the local context before implementing these kinds of social programs. If the state experts had asked what the local community needed, we could have shown them empirical evidence of our needs. We had community coalitions and epidemiologic evidence that demonstrated

---

1. https://prevention.nih.gov/research-priorities/dissemination-implementation/Evidence-based-practices-programs.

precisely what we needed to do to reduce HIV transmission in our jurisdiction. As Guba (cited in Stringer 1999: xi–xii) writes,

> We have witnessed, during the past half century or so, determined efforts to find general solutions to social problems, be they low pupil achievement, drug abuse, alcoholism, AIDS, or other challenges. The cost to national economies has been prodigious, and there is precious little to show for it. . . . Without intimate knowledge of local context, one cannot hope to devise solutions to local problems. All problems are de facto local; inquiry must be decentralized to the local context.

Community-based action research is one way to avoid this sort of pitfall, and it is an excellent way for academic researchers to be involved in local communities. It leverages the knowledge and skills of the researcher alongside the knowledge and skills of the people who benefit from community health interventions.

When planning any type of community-level intervention, consider using community-based action research as a tool for bringing community members together, identifying the *real* problem, and creating a workable solution.

This method flips traditional research on its head. Instead of a researcher coming into a community, extracting information, and then leaving, with this method community members conduct research and implement programs themselves. The researcher acts as a guide who teaches them how to use the tools. In this way, community members are empowered to identify what *they* believe are the most important concerns to tackle and they learn how to be effective at solving other problems in the future, without need of the researcher. A sustainable model is put in place to strengthen community resilience.

Community-based action research emerged out of the "participatory turn" in social science (Harper and Gubrium 2017: 5). Gullion and Tilton (2020: 20) note that

> this "turn" itself arose out of a critique of social science (anthropology specifically) as the product of Western colonialist thinking that tended to situate the (Western, white) researcher into an objective expert and people under study into passive objects. The participatory turn demands that people be seen as experts on their own experiences, that assumptions about scientific objectivity and truth be questioned, and that people be active participants in any research undertaken in their communities.

Let's look at how this is done.

Implementing a Community-Based Action Research Project

Mulrennan, Mark, and Short (2012: 246) write that in a community-based action research project,

> (1) the community defines and drives the agenda; (2) the community is involved in all phases of the research with active measures to reallocate power and ensure

reciprocal transfer (co-learning) of knowledge, skills, and capacity; and (3) research outcomes should benefit all parties, with the community receiving tangible and practical benefits as a result of their participation, in forms that advance social change and social justice.

One of the initial tasks in community-based action research is to bring together community members who are interested in working together to address a need in their community. This group should create a social map of the community. Consider variables such as age, gender, race, ethnicity, social class, income, religion, language, ability, sexuality, and so on. Marginalized groups in one community may not be marginalized in another, and marginalization may be occurring outside of traditional demographic categories. You want to ensure that all the various groups that are impacted by the need are represented in your working group. It's important to keep the working group thinking about who they might be missing and for it to find people who can act as the voice for the various impacted groups.

The definition of who is underrepresented varies based on the demographics of the community. Therefore, you need to understand who makes up that community so that you can identify who, if anyone, is missing from your working group. Not only does the absence of people from your group mean you're missing important information but also when people discover they have been left out (even when this happened by accident), they may create hostility and negativity in the community about what your group is working toward.

In his work on people living with disabilities, James Charlton coined the phrase "nothing about us without as" (cited in Strega and Brown 2015: 3). By this, he meant that social policies should not be created for people living with disabilities without their input. We can broaden this idea to fit other groups—don't make plans for people who aren't invited to give you input. In my own hometown, people who speak Spanish should be included in any community project. There are also many Vietnamese speakers in my community. There is a town within a thirty-minute drive from me where a researcher would want to include Hindi and Chinese speakers because of the large numbers of immigrants who have settled there. Another consideration for research in my community would be to include stay-at-home moms and homeschoolers if the project calls for it—my community has a sizable population of them, which has grown since the COVID-19 pandemic began. After schools reopened, some families decided homeschooling worked better for their children and chose not to send their kids back to school. That may not be the case in other communities. For this community, this is good information to have. If a group wanted to distribute health information through the schools, it would miss these families.

As with other types of qualitative inquiry, gatekeepers can be of tremendous help to you. A gatekeeper is someone who can give you entrance into a community. They can introduce you to people and validate your presence. They are a trusted person in the community who can let others know they can trust you.

In this type of research, finding a gatekeeper is not as daunting as it might first seem. They are usually already active

If someone claims to be a spokesperson for a particular group, ensure that they really are qualified to do so.

with building bridges between groups. Ask different groups in the community. Who speaks for this group? Who is trusted to speak for the group? Who knows people in this group? Sometimes community health workers will serve in this role. You can also look to alternative or nontraditional healers. Sometimes a veterinarian will serve in this capacity (this is especially true for research in rural areas). At the same time, if someone claims to be a spokesperson for a particular group, ensure that they are actually qualified to do so. I was once part of a community group in which an employee from a local health department continually spoke on behalf of single mothers. She was an excellent advocate, but she wasn't a single mother herself and she did not understand what it was like to be a single mother. In this case, it would be helpful to include both the health department employee—who could provide a broad overview of the community—and a single mother who is active in the community. The single mother would bring knowledge of the lived experience of what it is like to be a single mother and the needs of single mothers.

Once you have pulled together a representative group of community members, you can focus on the needs of the community and possible interventions. Community-based action research allows us the opportunity to custom design health interventions for our own communities, which in turn increases the likelihood that the programs will be successful.

People are experts on their own lived experiences. If you ask people what they need, they often know the answer; they are just unable, for whatever reason, to get what they need. It's important to ask the question because the answer often does not align with what outside experts think people need.

I worked in a large disaster shelter following Hurricane Katrina. All of the experts had their own agendas as to what should be done for the people who came to the shelter, and they did not coordinate with each other. Leaders from the school districts wanted to get the children enrolled in school as quickly as possible. The people running the shelter thought that finding families more permanent housing was most important. Both groups set to task to get these things done as quickly as possible. Meanwhile, my colleagues and I spoke to people and asked them, "What do you need right now?" One person said eyeglasses. They had lost their glasses and wanted to take care of that before worrying about anything else. Another person said she needed help locating her cousin. To be sure, housing and school were important and needed to be taken care of, but they were not pressing issues for the people who had just been through a major disaster. Their basic needs and concerns needed to be addressed first, before they were asked to make higher level decisions. In a traumatic situation, this is where we should begin. Get the woman some glasses so that she can see. Not having them caused an additional stressor for her; getting the glasses would ease some of her trauma response and help her move to her next need, which might indeed be housing or school for her children.

Your Role as Researcher

Because of its collaborative approach, community-based action research feels different from researcher-led projects. In most academic research training, the researcher is the clear leader of the project. This is with good reason—the researcher is the expert. In community-based action research, however, that role is flipped. The community members are the experts. The researcher helps them when they need help and gets out of the way when they don't need help.

A public health department director once told me that people don't know what they need—that they need an expert to tell them. That was a terrible attitude to bring into public health practice. People are experts on their lives. When people have a problem, they usually know what would fix their problem, but they might not have the knowledge or the resources to make that correction. This is where you come in. You help them get that knowledge and/or resources for themselves.

As you begin this type of work, take an assessment of your own skills, strengths, and weaknesses. Some of your skills are obvious. If you've been an instructor, you can probably speak to a large, diverse group of people without any problem. You probably already know how to facilitate meaningful conversations among people. You have been (or are being) trained in the nuts and bolts of research—how to write a research question, how to measure concepts, how to administer interviews and focus groups and surveys and other data collection techniques. You know (or are learning) how to analyze all sorts of data. You can write reports and scholarly papers. You can propose policy changes based on the results of your analytic work. You can meet with officials—your education gives you clout and the social capital to meet with people and be in spaces that others in your group may be excluded from. You probably have all sorts of other skills you can share as well.

Also, be honest with yourself about your weaknesses. If you aren't skilled at speaking in front of a large audience, find someone else who can take that role when it is needed. There is no expectation that you do everything; in fact, that would be counter to the collaborative ethos of community-based action research.

A good icebreaker early on in the project is to have everyone list their skills and strengths and share them with the group. Keep a record of these so that you know who to approach as different needs arise. You should distribute the labor so that everyone feels they are contributing to the project. That also gives people a sense of ownership and pride about the project. Keep in mind that community-based action research is

collaborative;
nonhierarchical;
inclusive; and
democratic.

A few years ago, I was invited to participate as a member of a community coalition that was working with our local school district on plans for responding to a mass shooter in the schools. School district officials hosted our first meeting at their facility, in a large conference room. There were approximately sixty people in attendance, representing many facets of community life. In addition to school district officials, there were representatives from the police department, fire and emergency medical services, the city emergency management, public health, the parent–teacher–student association (PTSA), the juvenile justice system, and a few nonprofit organizations. This was a nice mix of people with different perspectives on the issue, who could collaborate to write the district's active shooter plan.

Approximately ten minutes into the discussion, one of my fellow professors took over the conversation. He led it as if he were leading a class discussion. He called on people and asked them for input, he brought up great points, and occasionally summarized what we were doing. He's an excellent teacher, and he used his skills in this capacity.

The problem, however, was that we were not in a classroom, and these were working professionals, not college students. We were invited to the meeting to listen and offer our insight, not to lead the discussion. When he took on that role without being asked to, my colleague created a false hierarchy between himself and the other participants. In a community-based action research project, we need to avoid this. We should not be the lead.

Before embarking on this type of project, you need to decide if you are comfortable in that role. Are you ok with stepping aside and letting the process unfold as it will? If you prefer to direct the project, this might not be the right research method for you.

Finding Projects

Once you decide you're interested in conducting a community-based action research project, you will find there are no shortages of opportunities. Get involved with what is happening in your local community (or the community in which you would like to work). If you are having trouble getting started, look to the following (Gullion and Tilton 2020):

1. Nonprofit organizations
2. Local government
3. School boards/PTSAs
4. Hospitals
5. Local media

Let's consider each of these in more detail. Most (if not all) nonprofit organizations are required to collect and analyze data. They need information that shows funders that their work is impactful and that they know how to work with the local community. You can lend a hand in that regard. Often, nonprofits are predominately staffed by volunteers. Many would welcome assistance. They might appreciate working together to assess their programs or to conduct a needs assessment of your community. There may be interventions you could design and implement together. Reach out to the director of the organization, let them know your skill set and your willingness to help. You might consider signing on as a volunteer to better understand the organization's needs.

Local government is a great place to uncover unmet needs. Attend your city council or commissioner's court meetings or the meetings of any other governmental body in your community. At those meetings, you can both learn what the officials consider to be important and hear what concerns the residents bring forward. As you get to know the issues, you can begin introducing yourself and learn how you might help. Often, this is a way to find grassroots organizers who are working on local problems. Indeed, when I conducted my ethnographic study on natural gas drilling activism (Gullion 2015), this is how I began. I attended public meetings and identified who the prominent players were in grassroots activism. I then simply introduced myself to them, explained that I was a researcher interested in learning more about this topic, and asked if they would be interested in speaking with me about their experiences. School boards and PTSAs similarly have regular meetings, and by attending them consistently, you can learn what challenges the schools are facing.

Like nonprofit organizations, hospitals that receive federal funding are required to gather data about the local community and to implement community outreach. Their health educators would probably welcome your assistance.

Finally, make sure that you pay attention to local media, whether it is a traditional news source such as the local newspaper, blogs written about happenings in your town, or other media sources. Learn what people in your area are concerned about, and find places where you could lend your skills to help. Once you get involved in local events, you will find many opportunities for community-based action research projects.

Putting Theory into Action

There are several stages to a community-based action research project. First, you want to gather a group of people together who are interested in tackling a particular community problem. Together, you will define the goals of the project and what outcomes the group hopes to achieve. Next, you will work as a group to map the problem and gather data. You will use that information to decide what approach would be best to reach your goal and implement some sort of action.

Think broadly about who should be invited to participate in the group. These are your stakeholders. They are people who live in the community who have some sort of investment in the problem and who may be able to implement solutions to the problem. They can include the following:

- Residents
- Representatives from/of minority groups
- Elected officials
- Government officials
- Business owners
- Nonprofit organizations
- Hospitals
- School districts
- Churches
- Opinion leaders
- Clubs
- Social service organizations
- "Nonlegitimate" groups (e.g., gangs and motorcycle clubs)
- Others

Once you have gathered the group together, talk about what you all would like to achieve. Define your goals. When you are doing this, put in place both long-term and short-term goals. Discuss the steps needed to reach those goals, and decide what information your group needs in order to address this problem.

Mapping the Problem and Collecting Data

Mapping the problem and collecting data comprise the research piece of community-based action research. In community-based action research, you "will be engaging in systematic investigation that leads to social change" (Gullion and Tilton 2020: 88).

By mapping the problem, your group will be able to identify areas in which it can intervene. Remember that interventions don't have to be grand changes; small interventions can have a major impact on people's lives.

Several years ago, a friend of mine was riding bikes with her family in her neighborhood and nearly got run over by a car. They weren't on a major street; there was plenty of room for both vehicles and bikes. She was upset, and she mentioned it to several of her friends. As they talked about this, they agreed that the town really needed some bike lanes. They decided to do something about it. She worked to pull together a group of people who biked around town and others who were concerned with bike safety. This included owners of bicycle shops as well as parents.

Their first question was, What is happening here? Demanding that bike lanes be put throughout the town seemed untenable. They decided that the cost for that would be too high and that the city council would probably not support it. They began to map the problem. They narrowed their thinking down to vulnerable populations who are likely to ride bikes and to the areas those bikes would be ridden. They decided to scout out the streets around elementary schools because many children ride their bikes to school. This seemed like a good place to start. Who wouldn't agree that children should be kept safe while riding their bikes?

Next, they gathered data. They put out a call through their social networks to parents of elementary school children to help them map the problem. Together, they took photos of the streets around elementary schools to show areas where bike lanes could be implemented with a paint stripe, and they marked areas that bicyclists should be directed away from because it would not be safe to put in a bike lane without widening the road. They contacted groups that maintain records about vehicle/bicycle collisions and records about child injuries and deaths. This included auto insurance companies, state agencies, and the local medical examiner. They plotted those events on a street map of the town. They also spoke informally to workers at bike shops around town to get their perspective; the bike shop owners knew about many dangerous routes that should be avoided.

They then presented their data to members of the school board and asked if the members would join their cause. Many of the members did. The group invited the school board members to present the data to the city council because the school board had more social capital and clout than the parents alone. The fact that the school board was involved generated local media interest, which the group of parents may not have been able to get otherwise. Together, school officials and parents presented their data to the city council and asked that the city create bike lanes around the schools.

Cities are bureaucracies, and change takes time. The council members decided that the city should do its own investigation of the problem, and they created a task force to deal with it. They invited my friend, the one who initially started all this, to serve on the task force, along with one of the school board members. The task force reviewed the data the parents collected, and it brought in additional data the city maintained about traffic patterns and flow. The task force sketched out where it would be most cost-effective as well as most impactful to place bike lanes. It also created a plan to phase in bike lanes throughout the city over a number of years, which would include streets that would need to be widened to accommodate the lanes. As a stopgap measure, the task force proposed the creation of road signs that indicated that six feet should be given for bicycles where no lanes were present. During the course of their work, city officials expressed concern for streets in an area of town where day workers gathered to seek jobs. Many of the day workers rode bicycles to that area. They added plans for bike lanes in that area as well. The task force took their plan to the city council, which approved it.

In this example, we see that the community members were engaged to create social change in their city. They compiled compelling evidence, solicited community partnerships with people who had significant social capital (the school board members), and presented their case to city leadership. The media picked up the story and published articles about the idea. Community members stayed engaged and worked with city leadership on a plan for implementing this change. This took time and energy, and the change didn't happen overnight, but it did happen.

When you work with your own coalitions, brainstorm about where your group can get data about the problem it wants to address. Collect ethnographic data. Go to the places you're concerned about, see what it is like to inhabit those spaces. Collect demographic data. This can come from secondary data sources, such as the census or surveys conducted by governmental agencies. If you have access to community survey data, use that (if you can collect your own, even better). Learn about the community and this problem online. Consider news reports, blogs, neighborhood discussion groups, and so on. Review transcripts or minutes of public meetings (e.g., city council or other agencies) that have discussed your issue. Your group can also collect primary data through focus groups, interviews, and other data collection techniques. The data, and your analysis of them, will help guide your group on how to best respond to the issues. The data can also be used as evidence to support your case before policy builders, elected officials, and even used in a lawsuit if your group decides to take that route.

Conflict Management

When bringing a diverse group of people together to work on a common goal, conflict is inevitable. People will have different ideas on what the group should accomplish or different ideas about how to accomplish those goals. Although community-based action research is a noble endeavor, I'd be remiss if I didn't note how messy the process can be.

As you begin this type of research, you should be prepared for how you will manage conflicts. Many groups spend some time during their first meeting coming up with "ground rules" for the members. That is an excellent time to discuss how group members will address conflicts that arise. Talk about things such as the following:

1. How will you arrive at decisions?
2. Will you vote?
   a. Will the majority always win?
   b. Will that impinge on the rights of a minority group?
3. What if one or more members of the group dominate the conversation?
4. What if a group member bullies other members?
5. How will you add and/or remove members if needed?
6. How will you communicate (e.g., in-person meetings, online meetings, or through an asynchronous app)?

You also need to consider how to build the trust of all of the group members in you. People will come in with preconceptions about professors. Currently, there is a lot of anti-intellectual sentiment in popular culture, and some people may view you from that lens. Others might come to the group with previous experiences of researchers working in your community (especially if the project is being done in a college town). Those experiences will also color their opinion of you. Be clear with everyone in the group why you are there and how you would like to contribute. Although you might think you have a clear answer to the problem, set that aside. Engage in a lot of active listening before you jump in with your own ideas about what should be done.

Consider the perceptions people form about how you interact with the group members. It can be helpful to rotate who you sit by at the group meetings. This will help counter the perception that you are aligned with any individual or contingent. Also make sure that you help the group stay on task, and don't take sides in conflicts.

It's also important to stop and celebrate when you do accomplish something as a group, even small accomplishments. Thank people for the work they are doing, and show that you appreciate everyone in the group for taking time out of their lives and helping out. Making social change is not easy, and steps such as this will help when the group becomes discouraged and will help keep morale up.

What if People Don't Want to Participate?

As a parent, I'm frequently asked to volunteer for different organizations on behalf of my children. I've done my time in Cheer Boosters and Choir Boosters. I've helped lead field trips to museums and given guest talks. I've baked cookies (and bought them already made) for an assortment of fundraisers, and I've donated to all sorts of causes. But there's only so much time and energy I can give, and for as many things I've volunteered for, there were at least twice as many opportunities to give my time.

I have a full-time job with variable hours. I have friends and family. I have personal interests and hobbies. Although there are all sorts of causes out there that I believe in, I don't have time to give to everything. I am also frankly not interested in spending all my time in that way.

And that's ok. Most people are in similar situations.

When we are talking about community-based action research, we must keep in mind that the people we are working with are often volunteers. They are not receiving compensation for this work, and it is being done during their free time.

Some of the people most impacted by the problem you are working on won't be able to help. They may not want to help. And the people who do help may come and go. They may get caught up in other things and lose interest in the project. *Don't assume, however, that people are not participating because they don't care.*

There are all sorts of ways that people can be involved, so keep that door open wide. Maybe they can't give time but they can donate money or supplies to the group. Maybe the timing of your meetings or the location where you hold them make them inaccessible to some people. When people choose not to participate, be kind about it. Invite them to join anytime in whatever way they can. Ask them why they aren't taking part. Their answer may help you accommodate them.

Think about the ways in which your group may be inadvertently creating resistance to your project. Stringer (1999: 47) notes that

> when we try to get people to do anything, insist that they must or should do something, or try to stop them from engaging in some activity, we are working from an authoritative position that is likely to generate resistance.

Remember that people are busy, and be as inviting as possible while also understanding that it is ok if they choose not to participate in your project.

My daughter's cheerleading team used to sell T-shirts at football games to raise money. Well, the kids didn't do it, their parents did. They never brought in much money from the sales, and no one wanted to sit at the table selling shirts during the game. Parents wanted to be in the stands watching their kids perform.

The officers of the booster club ended up doing most of the work, and they got frustrated that other parents wouldn't help. Finally, someone asked why we didn't want to sell the shirts. In addition to missing out on watching their children perform, it was a pain to bring all the boxes of shirts to the game, cart them into the stadium, and set up the booth.

We brainstormed to find a fundraiser that would be easier on everyone. We decided to do an online fundraiser. Using a specialized app, the cheerleaders asked families and friends to donate money for particular items the squad needed, such as a set of new uniforms and money to cover costs for kids whose parents couldn't afford for them to cheer. This way, the team could be made up of kids with talent rather than comprising only wealthy kids.

In two days, the squad raised $16,000, which was much more money than the squad ever had in its account. The average balance was more like $1,000 for the year from selling shirts. Everyone was astounded. People who couldn't (or didn't want to) participate in the other fundraisers could just give some money, however much they wanted to. Because the fundraiser was online, the kids could easily contact everyone in their social networks. Individual donations ranged from $1 to $1,000 that someone's grandparents donated.

If you are not getting the participation you'd like, change your approach. And make it as easy as possible for people to participate.

Putting Action into Action Research

Community-based action research by definition contains an action component. This is not like other research where you conduct some inquiry and write up the results and then are finished. Your group is conducting research together for some purpose outside of your academic activities. As Gaudry (2011: 125) writes, "Research reports, even if inflammatory, damning, or enlightening, do not in and of themselves create action, and researchers often assume that knowledge creation and community-based action are the same." What will your action be? Although a research report can certainly be one of the outcomes, your group should brainstorm ideas for action. Gullion and Tilton (2020: 134) offer the following ideas:

1. Host a protest rally.
2. Conduct storytelling sessions.
3. Present about the problem at a city council meeting and ask for assistance.
4. Contact your elected officials and ask for intervention.
5. Write a technical report to educate officials and residents about the issue.
6. Write editorials about the problem for your local newspaper (letters to the editor work too).
7. Create fliers or posters about the issue and hang them around town.
8. Hold a town hall meeting.
9. Present at church groups, PTSA meetings, and other community organizational meetings.
10. Write an article for a magazine or blog.
11. Give a workshop on the issue. Or hold a conference.
12. Testify in court cases related to the problem.
13. Create art and display it around town.
14. Create and perform a play.
15. Create and distribute zines.
16. Tweet about it.
17. Hold a sit-in.
18. Circulate a petition with your demands.
19. Host a knit-in.
20. Host a march.

21. Picket relevant buildings.
22. Paint a mural (with permission).
23. Hold group work days.
24. Write and perform poetry.
25. Write and sing songs.
26. Write policy and give it to local elected officials.
27. Propose legislation.
28. File a lawsuit.
29. Make a film about the problem and show it at venues in town.
30. Hold a vigil.

There are many other activities your group may want to consider. As you brainstorm, think about the processes and the barriers that are in place for your action. For example, there may be rules in your community about where and what times you can legally picket, or how to go about speaking during a city council meeting. Although I don't advocate your group do anything illegal, if you decide to do so, make sure that you understand what the consequences will be. Have an attorney on standby who can help if any member of your group is arrested or runs into other legal issues because of their actions in the group.

Community-based action research is difficult work. You will be bringing a diverse group of people together, who may have very different ideas about how to proceed. They may also come together with their own baggage from previous attempts to work on this problem. Keep your expectations about outcomes reasonable. Focus on community-building while you work to meet your specific goals. Sometimes the process of bringing communities together and empowering people to work on their own behalf is a goal well earned (Mulrennan et al. 2012). The process is just as important, if not more so, than the outcome when it comes to community-based action research.

References

Gaudry, Adam J. 2011. "Insurgent Research." *Wicazo Sa Review* 26, no. 1: 113–136.

Gullion, Jessica Smartt. 2015. *Fracking the Neighborhood: Reluctant Activists and Natural Gas Drilling.* Cambridge, MA: MIT Press.

Gullion, Jessica Smartt, and Abigail Tilton. 2020. *Researching with: A Decolonizing Approach to Community-Based Action Research.* Leiden, the Netherlands: Brill.

Harper, Krista, and Aline Gubrium. 2017. "Visual and Multimodal Approaches in Anthropological Participatory Action Research." *General Anthropology* 24, no. 2: 1–8.

Mardiros, Marilyn. 2001. "Reconnecting Communities Through Community-Based Action Research." *International Journal of Mental Health* 30, no. 2: 58–78.

Moxley, David P., and Olivia G. M. Washington. 2013. "Helping Older African American Homeless Women Get and Stay out of Homelessness: Reflections on Lessons Learned from Long-Haul Developmental Action Research." *Journal of Progressive Human Services* 24, no. 2: 140–164.

Mulrennan, Monica E., Rodney Mark, and Colin H. Short. 2012. "Revamping Community-Based Conservation Through Participatory Research." *The Canadian Geographer* 56, no. 2: 243–259.

Reid, Sandra D., Rhoda Reddock, and Tisha Nickenig. 2014. "Breaking the Silence of Child Sexual Abuse in the Caribbean: A Community-Based Action Research Intervention Model." *Journal of Child Sexual Abuse* 23: 256–277.

Strega, Susan, and Leslie Brown. 2015. *Research as Resistance: Revisiting Critical, Indigenous, and Anti-Oppressive Approaches*, 2nd ed. Toronto: Canadian Scholars' Press.

Stringer, Ernest T. 1999. *Action Research*, 2nd ed. Thousand Oaks, CA: SAGE.

Further Reading

Foster, Jennifer, Sarah Gossett, and Rosa Burgos. 2015. "Improving Maternity Care in the Dominican Republic: A Pilot Study of a Community-Based Participatory Research Action Plan by an International Healthcare Team." *Journal of Transcultural Nursing* 23, no. 3: 254–260.

Shadowen, Noel L., Nancy G. Guerra, Ryan Beveridge, and Elizabeth K. McCoy. 2020. "A Resilient Research Approach: Using Community-Based Participatory Action Research in a Rural Area of India." *Journal of Community Psychology* 48, no. 8: 2491–2503.

Discussion Questions

1. What is community-based action research? How does it differ from other research techniques?
2. What ethical concerns might a researcher have when doing community-based action research?

Active Learning

1. Find out what concerns people in your local community have. Attend a city council meeting, school board meeting, or a meeting of some other governing body. Take notes on what issues were brought up.
2. Look for community discussion groups online. Document the concerns residents express.

Mindfulness Exercises

1. How could you work with your local community to create social change?
2. Do you have to be the leader of a project, or could you be in a supporting role? What might that look like for you?

8

Medical Narratives and Narrative Interviewing

Medical narratives include the stories of both patients and health care workers. In this chapter, we discuss how to capture and write those stories. This includes a variety of techniques, such as leading workshops for people to write their own narratives. We consider the power of storytelling and how to write stories that are compelling. We also discuss visual storytelling through the use of photovoice.

In his award-winning book, *Autobiography of a Disease*, Anderson (2017) writes about his experience with an infection, from the point of view of the bacteria that nearly killed him. He pulled the story both from his own fragmented memories and from his mother's notebook. His mother kept detailed notes throughout his illness, filling her notebook with information about his symptoms, medications, interactions with health care providers, and so on. Of it, he wrote,

> The book was filled with hospital desiderate: temperature and blood pressure readings, quantities of pills and dosage times, the names of hospitalized conditions, medical license numbers, insurance contracts. She had chronicled weeks of her son's convalescence, a portrait in data of illness, but also an archive of not-knowing. (p. 14)

Anderson also researched his condition and inserted details to round out his narrative. Over the course of his tale, we also learn his backstory, Anderson's life before the illness, his family, his friends.

Such recordkeeping is a fantastic way to keep track of the details of the story. When my students say they would like to do this type of research, I advise them to immediately begin journaling. The journal is data.

Qualitative Research in Health and Illness. Jessica Smartt Gullion, Oxford University Press. © Oxford University Press 2024.
DOI: 10.1093/oso/9780190915988.003.0009

Writing medical narratives helps us to both tell the story of health and illness and make meaning from the experience. These can also be one form of autoethnography (which we discuss in more detail below). These stories help us understand the experience of illness, to have empathy with both patients and health care providers, and help frame the reader's own experience of health and illness.

Weaver-Hightower (2019: 3) writes about the process of writing an autoethnography about the stillbirth of his daughter:

> How do you convey a secret experience you know because you've *been there* and *done that*—to someone who doesn't know it? How do I tell my reader what my participant felt, believed, or did? What quotations tell that story? What themes? How do I get my readers to understand another way of being human?

Let's look at some ways to do just that.

Creative Nonfiction

Medical narratives use creative nonfiction to tell stories. In this section, we discuss how to write creative nonfiction. This is a very different skill than writing a scientific research report.

Humans are storytelling creatures. It is how we convey a lot of information to one another verbally. When I ask my husband how his day went, he will tell me a story about something that happened. If I ask my mom how her doctor's visit went, she'll tell me the story of the encounter. But although we tell each other stories every day, many of us have not been trained on how to write a good story.

Good stories have relatable characters, who want/desire something and have to overcome obstacles to get it.

Good stories have relatable characters, who want/desire something and have to overcome obstacles to get it (Hart 2011; Gullion 2022). They also have a narrative structure, called a story arc. The arc carries the reader through the story as it unfolds. You can think of this as a theorized plot (Golden-Biddle and Locke 2007: 4; Gullion 2022), as an invisible thread that guides your reader through your story. Visualize a story arc as a bell curve. According to Hart (2011), there are five major areas under the curve:

1. Exposition
2. Rising action
3. Crisis
4. Climax/resolution
5. Falling action/denouement

Nearly all good stories follow this arc, whether fiction or nonfiction. Pay attention to narratives you enjoy, and see if you can identify their story arcs. Along the curve are plot points—events that alter the trajectory of the action. Hart (2011: 10) writes, "A plot emerges when a storyteller carefully selects and arranges material so that larger meanings can emerge." This is what we want when we write medical narratives or autoethnographies—for larger meanings to emerge before our readers.

Let's look more closely at the different stages under the curve. The first is exposition. This is where we introduce our reader to the world we want them to see and give them just enough background to set up our tale. This section should not be too long or it will get boring (Don't you hate novels that take dozens of pages to get to the action?). In exposition, we set the scene and give the reader a reason to want to keep reading—to make them want to know what happens next. Here's an example:

Jenny didn't know that something was wrong with the baby. She held his slick, just-born body against her chest, and whispered, hello.

In two sentences, we have given the reader expository detail. A woman named Jenny has just given birth to a son. That is the scene. The passage also draws the reader in with a big unanswered question: What's wrong with the baby? (Gullion 2016).

The story should quickly move to the second area under the curve: rising action. Something needs to happen. The following is an excerpt from one of my own medical narratives for illustration:

"We need to talk about the spring," [my department chair] said.

Next spring would be my last semester as a graduate student; I planned on teaching and finishing up my dissertation. I was going to give birth in February, defend my dissertation in April, and graduate in May. Some of the other graduate teaching assistants had recently told me they'd already received their teaching assignments for the spring. I was currently the senior among them, and it was a general policy that seniority equated better classes. This fall I was teaching research methods and statistics, and so I assumed I would teach them again.

"I can't hire you as a GTA in the spring since you are pregnant," she said. "It would be too disruptive to have you leave in the middle of the semester." She picked some lint off her sweater, flicked it on the floor, and stared at me. (Gullion 2008: 17)

Here you can see some exposition—the paragraph about being a pregnant graduate student—which is followed by rising action—the department chair's announcement that I won't have a job because I am pregnant. The protagonist (me) is confronted with a problem (unemployment and loss of insurance benefits right before having a baby).

Indeed, the protagonist will often be confronted with a number of problems, which is good for keeping tension in the story. This tension helps pull the reader along through your narrative.

Hart (2011: 119) writes that "a story is a journey, and journeys can be tedious or fascinating." We've all read tedious writing. We want our story to be fascinating.

The forward motion of our story is called its pacing. It is how fast or slow the story moves. To portray movement, use action verbs to show what is happening. Gullion (2016: 35) notes,

> We can also make sure that we parcel out information and not give the readers the conclusion too soon. Give the reader time to imagine what is going to happen next and how the story will end; most readers enjoy a pleasant surprise when what they've imagined is not quite what happens.

As the tension builds, we reach the third section under the curve: the crisis. At the moment of crisis, "everything hangs in the balance" (Hart 2011: 34). The protagonist will either win or be crushed—we are biting our nails to find out. And then, climax, resolution. We learn the outcome. This is the fourth area under the curve, where the tension of the story dissolves and we learn what happens.

The last area under the curve is falling action. This is where you wrap up any loose ends. Just like exposition at the beginning of the story, don't spend a long time in falling action. "Wrap things up as quickly as possible and leave the stage" (Hart 2011: 39).

Hart (2011) suggests, and I agree (Gullion 2016), that you should end your story with a kicker. This is a line or phrase that locks up your story, yet leaves your reader wanting more. Editorial writers often employ this technique. Here's an example of one from my book, *Fracking the Neighborhood* (Gullion 2015). The book ends with a kicker that indicates this story is not over:

> As I was finishing this manuscript, activists in the city of Denton won a significant victory in their fight against urban natural gas activities, and Denton became the first city in Texas to ban hydraulic fracturing.
>
> A grassroots organization called the Denton Drilling Awareness Group amassed thousands of signatures on a petition calling for a ballot measure to ban fracking within the city limits. In November of 2014 the ban was put to a vote, in which it prevailed overwhelmingly despite an intensive pro-industry campaign. One pro-drilling organization, Denton Taxpayers, purportedly spent about $700,000 fighting the measure, using funds largely donated by natural gas companies (Heinkel-Wolfe 2014).
>
> In response to the outcome of the vote, the Texas Railroad Commissioner said that "he was disappointed that voters 'fell prey to scare tactics and mischaracterizations of the truth in passing the hydraulic fracturing ban'" (Baker 2014). Denton's mayor, on the other hand, defended the voters' choice and proclaimed that the city would "exercise the legal remedies that are available to us should the ordinance be challenged" (Baker 2014).
>
> While passing the ban, the voters of Denton also elected a slate of Republican candidates into office.
>
> A lawsuit challenging the ban was filed by noon the day after the vote.

The last line is the kicker. Although the book has come to an end, the story continues.

Show, Don't Tell

Show, don't tell, is a writer's maxim. Particularly in narrative writing, show your reader the happenings rather than telling them. Let's compare these two descriptions, both gathered from observations and interview transcripts (Gullion 2016: 65):

> Telling: The conditions at the county jail are deplorable.
> Showing: Joan wakes with a start—someone is pulling her hair. She reaches through the darkness to find a warm furry mass. She leaps from her bunk, squealing, disgusted. It's the third night in a row she's woken to rats chewing on her hair. Her bunkmates scream at her: "Shut the fuck up, bitch!" She lays back down on the concrete platform, puts her arm under her head as a pillow, and cries.

Do you see how much more powerful showing is? It's important with this type of research to practice showing the scenes and events to the reader. This also helps the reader draw the conclusions that you want them to make. Reading Joan's story would probably lead the reader to think the conditions at the jail are terrible, without my having to tell them that. The reader draws the conclusion that I want them to draw.

Geertz (1973) argues that we should engage in what he calls thick description to give the reader a sense of what it is like to be part of that phenomenon. This brings life to your writing. Thick description also provides evidentiary support for your analytic writing. With thick description, you become a storyteller.

One way to do this is to find compelling details in your data (e.g., the rats chewing on the prisoner's hair) that will catch your reader's attention. These details help draw the reader into the story and make them want to keep reading. Pay attention to what catches your attention, what details you notice, and use them in your writing. Some ideas for thick description include the following:

> What did the place look like?
> What did you smell while you were there?
> What sounds did you hear?
> Were you inside or outside? What was the temperature like?
> What made you comfortable or uncomfortable in that space?
> Describe the people you interacted with (without giving away identifying information).
> What did they look like?
> How did they interact with you?

Think about sensual details. Narayan (2012: 36) suggests that we "describe the emotional and bodily sensations of moving through a place." Was the room cold? Did it smell like bleach? Or lavender? Or lavender and bleach with an undertone of infection and a whiff of body odor? Were the nurses talking loudly at the nurses' station, or did they whisper? Did they seem happy or somber? Could you hear alarms going off in patients' rooms? Or the hum of an electric floor cleaner as a janitor polished the hallway? Was the plastic chair you sat in while you waited hard? Did it hurt your back?

To do this, you must have high-quality field notes. As Madden (2010: 152) writes, "Good writing springs from good data. Evocation, thick description, persuasion, and a nice turn of phrase are so much easier to accomplish when you've got the data organized and marshaled behind you." Show us the world in your writing.

You can also show the reader what is happening in your setting through the use of quotes and conversations. "If you want to tell a true story," Hart (2011: 129) writes, "your readers should hear your characters talk to one another." Quotes from your participants "lend authority, tell us what others think, and add colorful voices" to the tale (Hart 2011: 128). The following examples are from my book, *Writing Ethnography* (2016: 79–81).

There are many ways you can include your participants' words in your ethnography. Let's look at several together. In this example, I use one interview transcript and present it in different ways.

This is an interview I conducted with a woman I've given the pseudonym of Mallory. I begin with a simple summary of the transcript. It goes like this:

> Mallory said she first learned that natural gas wells would be drilled on her property from her neighbor. She felt like the drillers did not care about her well-being at all.

In that passage, I paraphrased Mallory's words from the transcript. Another way to write this up is to use an extended quote from the transcript:

> They came onto our neighbor's property on August 29, 2009, and that was a Saturday. And I was actually in the living room, working out on my elliptical. And I saw trucks starting to show up, and I thought, that's odd. And a few minutes later my neighbor called me and he said they're coming to put in a well, and there's nothing I can do about it.

This quote gives us more detail and lets the reader listen to Mallory's voice as she tells her own story. Now let's write a conversation. In the interview, Mallory relates a conversation that her neighbor had with representatives from the drilling company. This passage is still a direct quote from the interview transcript. Mallory described the conversation between the neighbor and a man from the natural gas drilling company during her interview:

> My neighbor walked up to the men parked by his pond. "Do you want to fish?" he asked. Because a lot of people come out here to fish, it's kind of a neighborly thing to let people fish your pond. A man got out of one of the trucks, looking apologetic. "I'm really sorry," the man said, "but I'm actually looking to see where I'm going to put my bulldozer."
> "What bulldozer?" my neighbor asked.
> "I'm sorry, we're . . . they're getting ready to put a gas well here."

We could also embed that conversation into a larger conversation between Mallory and the interviewer, again relying on the interview transcript for the exact wording of that conversation:

> Mallory recounts the conversation with her neighbor. "He walked up to the men parked by his pond. 'Do you want to fish?' he asked. Because a lot of people come out here to fish, it's kind of a neighborly thing to let people fish your pond. A man got out of one of the trucks, looking apologetic. 'I'm really sorry,' the man said, 'but I'm actually looking to see where I'm going to put my bulldozer.' 'What bulldozer?' my neighbor asked. 'I'm sorry, we're . . . they're getting ready to put a gas well here.'"
>
> "So it's on his property? Someone just shows up on his property?" I ask.
>
> Mallory nods. "It's like we're not even here."

Each of the above examples remains true to the transcribed conversation between Mallory and the interviewer; the examples are simply presented differently. All of them convey that same feeling as in the original summary: Mallory said she first learned that natural gas wells would be drilled on her property from her neighbor. She felt like the drillers did not care about her well-being at all. Our own creativity comes into the writing as we decide how to best present the information. If we wanted to play with the form a bit more, we could also write this scene as an ethnodrama:

Neighbor:	Do you want to fish? A lot of people come out here to fish.
Gas Driller:	I'm really sorry, but I'm actually looking to see where I'm going to put my bulldozer.
Neighbor:	What bulldozer?
Gas Driller:	I'm sorry, we're . . . they're getting ready to put a gas well here.

Or how about a poem?

> Standing by the pond,
> He asked the strangers
> Did they want to fish? No.
> We're looking for a place
> To put the bulldozer.
> *It's like we're not even here.*

We can be creative with how we choose to present the same information. As you can see, each form continues to maintain the original sense that the drillers are unconcerned with the residents' feeling about their well-being. You may want to play with several different lengths and forms to find which works best with the goals of your narrative—which form hits that point hardest, that important line of "it's like we're not even here"?

Another part of showing, not telling, is character development. In the above examples, we learned a little about Mallory, her neighbor, and the man with the bulldozer. We can think about the people we interact with as characters in the story of our research.

Our characters can be individuals, or we can create composite characters who stand in for a group of people with similar traits. A composite character would be a "typical case" in your project. If you are going to introduce composite characters into your narrative, you should alert your reader that you are doing so.

A danger of composite characters is relying on stereotypes who are flat and not terribly interesting. People are multidimensional, with both likable and flawed qualities. Make your characters come alive with action and details. "Character," Hart (2011: 76) writes, "is the key to reader interest. Ultimately, we define ourselves in terms of others. What we really want to know is what, how, and why human beings *do*." And who better to explain those doings than a social scientist?

Include descriptive details to help your reader imagine your characters. You don't have to include too much exposition; instead, you can tap into your readers' pre-existing frameworks and references so that they create their own image of your character. For example, if I tell you that John is a tall, scarecrow-thin man, with a wisp of a comb-over, you can probably picture a version of him. Your image may differ from mine, but that's ok. We are using him to represent a class of people. You can also include specific details to make your characters memorable. Perhaps John also has a large mole right next to his nose, and he often removes his glasses and cleans them with the shirt of his scrubs.

The Stories We Tell

When something happens to a person, they interpret and reinterpret the event through the stories they tell themselves and others. Stories, and thus memories and tellings, are not stagnant. When we interview people, we get different interpretations. Everything they tell us is subjective, filtered through their (ongoing) understanding of events.

As an example, we can think of stories people tell about critical events. While the September 11, 2001 (9/11) terrorist attacks were happening in the United States, people were already constructing a story about what was going on. Two weeks after the event (as they got more information), those stories shifted and evolved. A year after the event, people asked each other what they were doing when the attack happened. This became a norm that is practiced in the United States every year on the date of the anniversary. Even though that day is important to many of the people who lived through it, they lose details over time. Two weeks later, I probably could have told you what I was wearing that day. Today, I don't have a clue. The stories we tell also change with new information—twenty years of war later, my story of 9/11 is probably much different than the story I told that day. Yet social scientists treat interview data as Truth. We need to keep in mind that when we interview someone, we are hearing an interpretation of an interpretation.

All stories are influenced by the social events happening around the teller, both at the time of the event and at the time of the telling. "Individual life stories are very much embedded in social relationships and structures and they are expressed in culturally specific forms," Maynes, Piece, and Laslett (2008: 3) write, "Read carefully, they provide unique insights into the connections between individual life trajectories and collective forces and institutions beyond the individual."

As mentioned previously, journaling is an important component of narrative inquiry. Journal entries become invaluable data later, as we inevitably reinterpret events and forget detail. Narrative researchers often use documents such as journals, letters, emails, texts, medical charts, and other objects as data.

Maynes et al. (2008: 3) write,

> The stories that people tell about their lives are never simply individual, but as told in historically specific times and settings and draw on the rules and models in circulation that govern how story elements link together in narrative logics.

Narrative Interviewing

In narrative interviewing, the participant is invited to tell their story. The researcher asks questions, but these are more in-depth than other forms of interviewing. The participant and interviewer are literally having a conversation. The conversation is dialogic in nature.

I used this type of interviewing in my fracking project. Most interviews began with asking environmentalists the question, "How did you get involved in this?" For regulatory officials, the first question was something like, "What it is that you and your agency do?" (related to fracking). From there, we would have a conversation. There was no set questionnaire. This type of interviewing helps you build a story of a phenomena. It is not meant for comparing individuals to each other or deriving themes (although some commonalities might become apparent). Maynes et al. (2008: 6) note that

> individual stories are treated as interesting in and of themselves, but their analytic value rests on their ability to reveal something new about a social position defined by and of interest to the analyst but more legible through an insider's view.

Narrative research emphasizes research as relational (Butler-Kisber 2010). It requires that you have good rapport with your participant and that you are able to keep the conversation on topic. Narrative interviews are typically long and may be conducted over a number of sessions.

Butler-Kisber (2010: 78) also writes about four criteria that could be used to judge the quality of narrative research:

1. They are comprehensive, with ample evidence.
2. There is coherence between and among the parts of the story.
3. The narrative provides insight that resonates with the reader.
4. There is an aesthetic to the story; it is well-told.

Narrative interviewing can include life histories or oral history (stories surrounding a particular event). Narrative analysis can also be done of secondary data, including archival analysis.

Jordan (2020) conducted a multiyear project with artist Harold Stevenson. She interviewed him in his home many times and later in a nursing home. They became good friends, and he left her his archive when he died. This included boxes and boxes of documents, letters, paintings, photographs, designer clothing, and so on. The archive was so large that she had to rent a space to store it. Because she wanted to write a life history of Stevenson and pop art, she contacted his friends, museums that house his paintings, and others who could shed light on his place in art history.

Although the details of archival analysis are beyond the scope of this book, it is one way to conduct qualitative research. Most university libraries house archives. My own university houses a number of archives, including one on COVID-19 narratives, the Women Airforce Service Pilots official archive, and an archive of culinary arts and cookbooks dating back to the 1600s. Archives are a treasure trove of data and can be used to create a narrative about a person or event.

Photovoice

Another way to collect narratives of people's experiences is through a technique called photovoice or photo elicitation (Latz 2017). In this method, the researcher invites participants to take photographs and then explain the photos to the researcher.

Latz (2017: 43) writes that there are "three primary aims" to photovoice research:

(a) Encourage participants to document elements of their lives within their own terms; (b) raise levels of critical consciousness within the participants through critical dialog; and (c) reach policy makers with project findings to catalyze positive change, which will address the needs and/or issues identified by the participants.

This technique is usually informed by critical theory, with a social justice and social change orientation. When done well, it should empower the contributors to better advocate for their needs.

Typically, the participant is given a prompt and then invited to take photographs in response to that prompt. The prompt is driven by the research question. For example, if your research question is "How do teen mothers experience motherhood?" you could give the mothers in your study the prompt, "Take photos of what it feels like to be a teen mom." The participants are empowered to interpret that prompt how they see fit.

After they take the photographs, the participants are usually asked to choose one or two that they believe most accurately (or poignantly) represent their experience and then share those with the researcher. The quality of the photos as art is less important than the images the participants choose to capture. The researcher then interviews the participants about the photos they chose and uses both the interviews and the photos as data. The end result of photovoice projects is usually a photo essay and/or gallery showing, coupled with information from the interviews.

Latz (2017) identifies seven steps to photovoice projects:

1. Identification
2. Invitation
3. Education
4. Documentation
5. Narration
6. Data analysis
7. Presentation

We review these below.

As in any research project, the researcher must first develop a research question and conduct a thorough review of the literature. What is it that you wish to know? Coupled with that question, you should also ask who needs the information you will learn. Once you have identified your research question, you can write prompts for your participants to work with. The prompts should be open-ended and open to interpretation. Think about questions that begin with phrases such as "What it is like," "How does it feel," or "Show me . . . ." You could also ask participants to photograph their interpretation of words that are meaningful to them, such as cancer patient, anorexic, or wellness.

In many photovoice projects, you will be using purposive sampling. That is, you want to find people who would like to participate based on some characteristic of interest. Perhaps you are interested in the experience of cancer patients. You could recruit patients and ask them to document what it feels like to sit for hours in an infusion center, receiving chemotherapy. Maybe you are interested in how obstetricians who are on call 24/7 balance work with family life. You could invite them to document how it feels to be called in to work during a family event. Latz (2017) recommends that you oversample—begin with more people than you think you will need—to account for attrition. Some people will probably not finish the project, and you don't want to find yourself with too few participants.

Before they can go out and take photographs, you need to explain your project to your participants; review ethical guidelines with them; and ensure that they have the technology to take the photos, save them, and share them with you. Given the fact that most people have smartphones with cameras, you will probably not need to worry about supplying cameras, but make sure you have access to some in case there are participants who don't have them. Some researchers choose to give everyone a cheap disposable camera, although the quality of the images is likely to be poor.

Another consideration is manipulation of photos, including the use of filters and the addition of text or other images on top of the original. Will you allow that? Or would you prefer the photos not be manipulated? Be clear with your participants about what you want from them.

You need to decide with your Institutional Review Board how you are going to handle privacy issues. As part of your consent process, there needs to be an extra form that documents that you own or co-own the photos and have the right to use them in print, presentations, and gallery showings. If your participants are going to photograph other people, they will need to get a photo release form signed by those people in order for the photo to be used in print, presentations, or exhibitions. If you do not want to do that, you can ask that they only photograph objects or scenes without people or that when they do photograph people, they use software to blur the peoples' faces. This can produce interesting results. Once a student sent me a photograph of the controls on the chair that she sits in to receive her chemotherapy treatments. There were buttons for heat and for different types of massages. She said that if it weren't for "the bag of toxic chemicals" hanging from her arm, it would be like she was getting her toenails painted.

You should also consider ahead of time what you will do if participants photograph something illegal. There could be ramifications of your use of those photos. You should discuss this issue with your participants during the consent process.

After the participants have taken their photos, the researcher will ask them to choose one or two that best represent their response to the prompt. The researcher will then interview the participants about those images. This is the narration phase of the project. The researcher will ask questions such as, Why did you choose this image? What is the meaning behind the images? The interview should be conversational rather than scripted. Talk about any manipulation they did to the photo. What filter(s) did they use and why? Did they add text or additional images to the main image? Why did they choose to do that?

Some researchers will also hold focus groups that include all of the participants in the study. The participants will be invited to view all the images and then have a group discussion about what they saw. The researcher should ask them to describe what they see. What resonated with them when they saw all the photos together? What do they think about them? Like the individual interview, this should be an organic process.

As in any project, you should keep field notes and analytic memos throughout the process. In terms of analysis, you can analyze the interviews, focus groups, and the photos. In Chapter 9, we discuss how to perform that analysis.

Finally, you need to decide how you will show the photos. A gallery exhibition to which all the participants are invited, and can invite whomever they want, can be gratifying and cathartic for all involved.

To give you a sense of how powerful this can be, I discuss a Masters of Fine Arts final project that I had the honor of taking part in.

Despite being a visual arts major, the student took my qualitative methods course to learn how to conduct interviews. She planned to do a photovoice project as her major exhibition for her degree.

For her project, she traveled to Iraq, where an American gatekeeper could help her set up interviews with women to discuss their daily lives. She wanted to know what it was like for women to live in a region that has been involved in wars for most, if not all, of their lives. How does one live daily life under those conditions?

The student did not speak Kurdish, the native language of the women in her study, so she found an interpreter. She then found seven women interested in taking part in the project. She went to their homes and interviewed them, and she took photographs of objects inside their homes and then talked to them about the images. The interviews were conducted through the translator, and they were audio recorded. Due to of the risk that the women could be killed for even taking part in the project, she chose not to photograph the women or anything that she thought would identify them.

She paid someone to transcribe the interviews verbatim and to translate them, so she had transcripts in both Kurdish and English. She then found another Kurdish speaker to listen to the recordings and check that the transcriptions were correct. Once that was verified, she deleted the recordings because she didn't want anyone to be able to identify the women's voices for safety reasons. She used the English translations for data analysis.

She wanted to do an exhibition in Iraq, but that was not feasible. Therefore, she held an exhibit in the United States. Her showing had seven stations in a large art gallery. On the wall in front of each station were photographs from each woman's home. Next to each photograph was a small box with a button the viewer could push to hear her interview read by someone else in Kurdish (again, this was to protect the participant's privacy and for possible safety concerns). A white table stood before each station. On it, she placed a book she had made with the English-only transcripts for viewers to read. She also placed objects of the type of things she had seen in the homes, such as certain types of tea or a shawl or other tactile objects. She wanted the exhibition to be as interactive as possible so that Americans could get a sense of daily life for Iraqi women.

As you read this, you might think about using the student's method for your own project. You may conversely be turned off from this method because it isn't peer-reviewed or evidence-based. Although that may be the "gold standard" in medical research, I hope you can see that there are other ways to get information about the world and other ways to understand people's experience. This can give new insight that can help us with treatment and healing.

Amplifying Marginalized Voices

It is not unusual for social scientists to say that they want to "give voice to the voiceless." This is an arrogant, savior mentality. Everyone has a voice, but people have different levels of access to amplify their voices. We don't give anyone voice, but we can amplify people's voices.

Maynes et al. (2008) argue that the use of personal narratives in the social sciences is a way to bring marginalized voices into the discussion. Through personal narrative, we can magnify details that would never otherwise be captured. We can find counternarratives to dominant narratives. We can counter slippery knowledge claims.

References

Anderson, Patrick. 2017. *Autobiography of a Disease*. New York: Routledge.

Baker, Max B. 2014. "Texas Town Bans Fracking in the Heart of Texas Oil Country." *Fort Worth Star-Telegram*. https://www.star-telegram.com/news/politics-government/article3906359.html.

Butler-Kisber, Lynn. 2010. *Qualitative Inquiry: Thematic, Narrative and Arts-Informed Perspectives*. Los Angeles: SAGE.

Ellis, Carolyn. 2007. "Telling Secrets, Revealing Lives: Relational Ethics in Research with Intimate Others." *Qualitative Inquiry* 13, no. 1: 3–29.

Geertz, Clifford. 1973. "Thick Description: Toward an Interpretive Theory of Culture." In *The Interpretation of Cultures: Selected Essays*, edited by Clifford Geertz, 3–30. New York: Basic Books.

Golden-Biddle, Karen, and Karen Locke. 2007. *Composing Qualitative Research*, 2nd ed. Thousand Oaks, CA: SAGE.

Gullion, Jessica Smartt. 2008. "Scholar, Negated." In *Mama, PhD: Women Write About Motherhood and Academic Life*, edited by Elrina Evans and Caroline Grant, 16–19. New Brunswick, NJ: Rutgers University Press.

Gullion, Jessica Smartt. 2015. *Fracking the Neighborhood: Reluctant Activists and Natural Gas Drilling*. Cambridge, MA: MIT Press.

Gullion, Jessica Smartt. 2016. *Writing Ethnography*. Rotterdam, the Netherlands: Sense Publishers.

Gullion, Jessica Smartt. 2022. *Writing Ethnography*, 2nd ed. Leiden, the Netherlands: Brill.

Hart, Jack. 2011. *Storycraft: The Complete Guide to Writing Narrative Nonfiction*. Chicago: University of Chicago Press.

Heinkel-Wolfe, Peggy. 2014, November 5. "Fracking Banned." *Denton Record-Chronicle*.

Jordan, Dian. 2020. *Art in the Community: The Harold Stevenson Collection*. Idabell, OK: The Museum of the Red River.

Latz, Amanda O. 2017. *Photovoice Research in Education and Beyond: A Practical Guide from Theory to Exhibition*. New York: Routledge.

Madden, Raymond. 2010. *Being Ethnographic: A Guide to the Theory and Practice of Ethnography*. Los Angeles: SAGE.

Maynes, Mary Jo, Jennifer L. Piece, and Barbara Laslett. 2008. *Telling Stories: The Use of Personal Narratives in the Social Sciences and History*. Ithaca, NY: Cornell University Press.

Narayan, Kirin. 2012. *Alive in the Writing: Crafting Ethnography in the Company of Chekhov*. Chicago: University of Chicago Press.

Weaver-Hightower, Marcus B. 2019. "Analyzing Self and Other in Autoethnography," In *How Qualitative Data Analysis Happens: Moving Beyond "Themes Emerged*," edited by Áine M. Humble and M. Elise Radina, 3–17. New York: Routledge.

Further Reading

Breny, Jean M., and Shannon L. McMorrow. 2021. *Photovoice for Social Justice: Visual Representation in Action*. Los Angeles: SAGE.

Luttrell, Wendy. 2020. *Children Framing Childhoods: Working-Class Kids' Visions of Care*. Bristol, UK: Bristol University Press.

Discussion Questions

1. How does narrative interviewing and writing differ from other approaches to collecting and writing about data? What are the advantages and disadvantages of this technique?
2. What is photovoice? When might you use it?

Active Learning

1. Write your own medical narrative. Think about a time you dealt with a health issue, or an encounter you had with a medical professional. Tell that story.
2. Give everyone in your class a prompt, such as "What does wellness mean to you?" and have the class conduct a photovoice project. Have each student take photographs and then choose the one that they believe best responds to the prompt. Show the images in class and let the class discuss them, like a focus group.

Mindfulness Exercises

1. What stories do you have about your own experiences of health and illness? Could any of those make for an autoethnography of the experience?
2. Go for a walk. Take photographs of how you are feeling.

PART III

Evaluation and Writing

9

Thinking with Data

There are many different ways of both managing and thinking with qualitative data. In this chapter, we explore a variety of analytic techniques, including coding, data mapping, grounded theory, and poetic inquiry. We also consider post-qualitative research and the ways in which post-qualitative inquiry posits additional ways of thinking with one's research phenomena.

Data Management

One of the major challenges for qualitative researchers is managing the sheer volume of data that are collected. When I was writing my book, *Fracking the Neighborhood* (Gullion 2015), I collected thousands of printed pages of text from interviews, blogs and other data from the internet, and posters and fliers. I had several notebooks filled with handwritten field notes and memos. I also had hundreds of photographs and both rendered and hand-drawn maps. And I had all of the literature I had read and consulted for the background and literature review. The sheer volume of materials was staggering.

Although most of the data were digital, I also collected all sorts of physical flotsam—fliers and other handouts, protest signs, bumper stickers, and a T-shirt. Weaver-Hightower (2019: 7) suggests researchers keep a "junk drawer" of materials. Will that T-shirt be relevant? Who knows? Maybe. Put it in the junk drawer. You could also photograph these items and add them to your digital repository of data.

Qualitative researchers are data hoarders, and you will need to find some way to organize your hoard. Software packages are available that can help you with this, and I recommend you try some to see if they work for you. I prefer to organize my data by hand, with

Qualitative researchers are data hoarders.

Qualitative Research in Health and Illness. Jessica Smartt Gullion, Oxford University Press. © Oxford University Press 2024.
DOI: 10.1093/oso/9780190915988.003.0010

colored notecards and piles for different topics. I maintain one main computer document in which I begin to write my notes and ideas. As I work through the data, I write my processes and findings there. That document can then be used to write a book or several journal articles.

I also keep a dedicated journal for the literature that I review. I start a new page with the reference for the piece and then take notes and write quotes that I think I might use (don't forget the page numbers!). This way, I have everything in one place instead of having to hunt for an article or book I've already read searching for information. I write by hand because that's what works best for me, but there is no reason why you couldn't do the same thing electronically. It would probably save time for you to do so because you could just copy and paste into whatever document you are working in.

I like to see what I am doing. When I get into the thick of data analysis, I use large sheets of presentation paper that can stick to the wall to map my data and draw a "big picture" overview of the project. I add sticky notes that can be moved around as needed until I have an understanding of how I want to present my findings.

Some people keep spreadsheets that document all of their materials with links to each item. Project management software can be useful for this as well; there are many systems available online, some of which are free.

Transcription

Once you have conducted your interviews, you want to put the data in a format for analysis. There are different ways you can do this. Traditionally, researchers transcribe their interviews into written text. We focus on transcription here, but note that some researchers use computer programs to code the audio directly rather than transcribing each interview. Some researchers just listen to the audio over and over and take notes.

Generally, you will want to transcribe interviews as soon as possible after the interview or event took place. There are several advantages to this. First, you will probably remember things that happened that you can take note of (e.g., facial expressions or body language), or analytic ideas may occur to you while you are working. Second, it ensures that you really *know* your data. This will make analysis easier because you are more readily able to remember who said what and when.

There are many transcription services available through the internet. If you choose to use one, make sure that it is used to doing academic transcription. Check for recommendations and ratings. Ask about rates (it can get expensive) and turnaround time. You will also have to get something from it certifying that it will keep your data confidential, and you need to make sure that your Institutional Review Board approves. Most services will have your completed transcripts back to you in a day or two. Make sure that you review all of the finished transcripts with the audio to ensure there are no errors.

Necessity breeds invention, and because so many things moved online during the COVID-19 pandemic lockdowns, transcription software has improved dramatically in order to make online gatherings ADA (Americans with Disabilities Act) complaint. Again, be sure to check the produced text against the interview; sometimes the results are far from what was said.

When I transcribe interviews, I build a table with three columns: speaker, text, and comments. If I plan to hand-code the data, I will include a fourth column called codes. Every time someone speaks, they have a new entry in the table. In the example shown in Table 9.1, the PI is the principal investigator (i.e., me). If you had multiple people conducting interviews for a project, you could number them or use some other identifier. For the participant (P), instead of using their real name, I use either a pseudonym or other code that only I and my research team (if I have one) know how to decode. This is done to protect confidentiality. If someone outside the research team were to somehow get their hands on the transcript, they would not be able to discern the identity of the participant.

The text is the verbatim dialog between us. I do not correct grammar or make any other changes to what was said. If I can't understand something that was said, I will write a note in brackets, such as [unintelligible] or [garbled]. If someone laughs or cries or makes other sounds, I put thoughts in brackets too, like this: [laughing], [snorts], [crying].

As I am transcribing, I jot down extra information in the comments section. For example, maybe I remember that the participant seemed uncomfortable with a question, or a waiter came over and interrupted us, or maybe as I am transcribing I think of how what

TABLE 9.1 Example of a Transcription

Speaker	Text	Comments
PI	How did you learn that they were going to do fracking on your property?	
P	I didn't know it was going to happen. My neighbor called me at work and said, they took down your fence and your horses are out.	
PI	What on earth?	
P	Yeah. They took apart my fence so they could drive their trucks in and I guess they cared less about my horses.	
PI	That sounds terrible.	
P	You can't imagine. I ran home and my neighbor helped me round up the horses, but I was like, what am I supposed to do with them?	There is a hitch in her voice—she seemed like she was going to cry, but she didn't.
PI	Because the fence was still down?	
P	Oh yeah. They never fixed my fence. In fact, I had to leave it open so they could come in and out.	Look up legality of this; see if they were supposed to have fixed it. Legal issues might be a relevant code.
PI	Is that even legal?	
P	Apparently, yes. They have to be allowed access to your property.	
PI	What did you do with the horses?	
P	I sold all but one. [starts crying] I stable her at a friend's barn. [crying]	

they said reminded me of something or that I should consider coding the data in a partic-ular way.

Beginning Data Analysis

While you may have conducted some preliminary data analysis already, once you have or-ganized your materials and transcribed audio and video files, it's time to get serious about data analysis. Analysis is not as linear as textbooks make it seem. You've probably been thinking about the data and writing analytic memos already.

> Throughout the process, researchers make ana-lytic moves.

By the time you reach analysis, you've already made a number of analytic moves. The first was deciding what to re-search and the best way to do that. The next was to name cer-tain objects "data" while leaving others out. Then you strived to capture those objects so that they would serve as analytic materials. Reading the literature relevant to your study constitutes another analytic move.

We should be transparent with our readers about how we performed our analytic work. To say that "themes emerged" and leave it at that, as researchers often do, puts analysis into a black box. Researchers often don't discuss their processes and procedures of analysis in nearly as much detail as they should (Humble and Radina 2019). The phrase becomes short-hand for analytic work. Perhaps this is partly why some people believe qualitative research is subjective—they are unfamiliar with the grit of analysis. Perhaps this is partly due to a lack of grammar to explain thinking; after all, that is what analysis entails. Thus, we read authors who "identified themes" in the data without an explanation of how that happens. Another issue that may come into play is the constraints of academic publishing. Most journals limit the number of pages allowed for an article, and the author(s) understandably wants to focus on the findings. If something is to be cut, discussion of analytic processes is a lot of text to chop. Unfortunately, "what is left is vague representations of qualitative analysis processes that offer little to the reader about the realities of what they look like' (Humble and Radina 2019: ix). This may explain why so many qualitative projects become books.

Qualitative analysis involves deep thinking about one's empirical materials, the in-formation one has gleaned, and the literature one has engaged. And although I can tell you about some of the tools that others have found helpful, ultimately *you must think*. And thinking—really thinking about these matters—is difficult. In most cases, there are no straight answers, no Truth with a capital T. Rather, there are interpretations of interpret-ations, which can be tentative and fleeting.

Sit with your data and think with them, using techniques in this book, others you've encountered, or even some you create on your own. If you do not do a deep dive into your data, if you do not get further than surface reading with minimal analytic backbone, your findings will be mundane at best. There are many ways to think with your data. But under-stand that done correctly, it is nonlinear, complex, and difficult to distill.

Thinking with our data allows us to make sense of the thousands of words/images/ objects that we have collected during the course of our research. We are not journalists; our goal is not to summarize events or just to tell a good story. Indeed, what makes the work academic is our analytic spin on it (I say this with no offense to journalists—many journalists do analytic work that I would consider to be academic as well, although their primary goal is usually to report events).

During analysis, we are trying to uncover larger meanings from our data, new insights and ways of thinking about the particular phenomena we're studying. In many cases, this involves tearing apart the narratives into smaller bits and reconstructing meaning from them. Charmaz (2014: 111) writes, "If you concentrate on taking fragments of data apart and asking what meanings you glean from these fragments, you will move into analysis." Deconstructing your data for analysis is not without criticism, however, as you will see later in the chapter when we discuss post-qualitative inquiry.

Coding

We begin with the most recognizable form of qualitative data analysis: coding. For this discussion, we are going to lean heavily on the work of Johnny Saldaña (2011, 2016). Saldaña (2016: 4) defines a code as "a word or phrase that symbolically assigns a summative, salient, essence-capturing, and/or evocative attribute for a portion of language-based or visual data."

Coding is a data-reduction technique, a way to make sense of the empirical materials you've collected. It can also help you write a written report of what you've found during the course of your research.

To code data, we examine every phrase and assign it a label. We then comb through the labels to see how they hang together, such that X [the phrase] is an example of Y [the code]. Codes are often written in vivo—that is, using the exact words of the participants. Let's code a small piece of text:

	Codes
Participant: I go to the barn once a week for my mental health. Working with the horses . . . even just brushing them. It's relaxing. I forget about everything else and it's just me and the horse. The physicality of the horse, the way the horse feels. Its movements, how it relates back to me. There's something magical about horse therapy.	Go to the barn Mental health Working Horse/Horses Brushing Relaxing Forget about everything Physicality Feels Movements Relates Magical Horse therapy

Once we've made a first pass through the data, we then take a second pass. Look back through the data and code at different intervals of text. This can be paragraphs, sentences, phrases, and individual words. This is all interpretive—what does the respondent *mean* when they said these things? Make multiple passes through the data, and begin collapsing the codes. For example, the codes "Mental health," "Relaxing," and "Forget about everything" could be examples of mental health effects of horse therapy. "Go to the barn," "Working," "Brushing," and "Relates" are examples of interacting with the horses. "Physicality," "Feels," and "Movements" are examples of the embodied experience of the therapy. The code "Magical" seems to stand on its own. It would be a good idea to look through the rest of the data to see if this word or others like it come up. It could be an interesting theme.

As you can see, we begin to find categories within our data that could be flushed out into themes. Just from this brief passage, we can see that this participant finds that the embodied experience of interacting with the horses leads to positive mental health effects. This example is brief. As we explore the totality of our data, we could see if this holds true for the other participants, and get more information about the horse/mental health connection.

Although coding is often associated with interview transcripts, we can code any analytic materials. This includes items such as news articles, blogs, photos, film/videos, and even your field notes.

As you code your data, I recommend you keep your research question handy (I tell my students to write it down and post it near their computer so it is easy to refer to). If you are thinking with a particular theorist, keep their work close as well. It can be easy to go down rabbit trails while coding. Although those trails may provide you with additional papers to write, they may also distract you from the goals you started the project with.

When I code interviews that are structured or semistructured, I begin by looking at the responses to my specific questions. This is a very basic first run through the data, but it gives me a sense of, or feeling for, the data across respondents.

Coding helps us recognize patterns in our data. As we code our data, we make multiple passes through it. In doing so, we identify larger categories that the codes imply. Categories can have a number of subcategories. Below, we discuss grounded theory, in which the researcher looks at relationships between/among categories.

It is important to note that the words "code," "categories," and "themes" are not interchangeable (Saldaña 2016). Rather, themes in the data are identified as the researcher collapses codes into categories that allow them to make assertions about what they found in the data.

Saldaña (2016: 5) writes that "coding is not a precise science; it is primarily an interpretive act." You and I might code the same data differently. This is why we keep records of how we create and employ our codes. It's helpful to create an electronic file or written journal that logs your process. This will prove invaluable when writing your methods and analysis sections in traditional research papers or thesis/dissertation work. Saldaña (2011: 46–53) argues for keeping analytic memos as you code. In these memos, you should reflect and write about the following:

1. Your code choices and their operational definition
2. The participants' routines, rituals, rules, roles, and relationships
3. Emergent patterns, categories, themes, concepts, and assertions
4. Possible networks and processes (links, connections, overlaps, flows) among the code's patterns, categories, themes, concepts, and assertions

5. An emergent or related existing theory
6. Any problems with the study
7. Any personal or ethical dilemmas with the study
8. Future directions for the study
9. The analytic memos generated thus far (meta-memos)
10. Tentative answers to your study's research questions
11. The final report for the study

Rosenblatt and Wieling (2019) argue that coding is subjective and therefore should be reviewed by multiple coders. For this reason, some projects involve a team of researchers. The researchers may want to code the data individually and then meet to discuss what each member found. In this case, they look for intercoder reliability—in other words, how well the findings match up among the coders. This technique can also be used to make a codebook to analyze additional data when dealing with very large data sets. A codebook is explicit instructions about how and what to code. Researchers create codebooks for consistency across cases as well.

> A codebook is explicit instructions about how and what to code.

Another way to code is to quantify qualitative data. It may be difficult to understand why one would want to collapse rich data into numerical data, but occasionally it can be a useful way to see the data in a new light. For example, researchers might count certain words or phrases to determine how prominent they are throughout the data. Word clouds help visualize the counts by increasing or decreasing the size of a word's proportionality to the number of times the word appears in the document (Figure 9.1). There are many free word cloud generators on the internet. Usually, they will let you discount small words such as "the" and "and."

Statistics are not usually a data analysis technique for qualitative researchers. Rather, we want to capture the richness of experience behind and beyond statistics. Numbers essentialize and create reality without troubling (or often even acknowledging) their derivation (Gullion 2018). Be mindful that changing words to numbers erases the beautiful, rich data you spent time collecting.

Some researchers choose to use a mixed methods approach, in which they use both qualitative and quantitative methods in their study. They use a variety of different methods to enhance the overall project. For example, a researcher might want to conduct a large, random sample survey and then invite participants to be part of an additional in-depth interview. Or a researcher might conduct interviews to help write the questions for a later survey project.

One problem that I have seen among my own students is that of overcoding. Rather than move into an analytic phase in which they understand what all those codes mean, and how they relate to each other, they just keep coding. They show me transcripts that are a hot mess of different highlighted colors and overlapping codes. As you do this work, it can

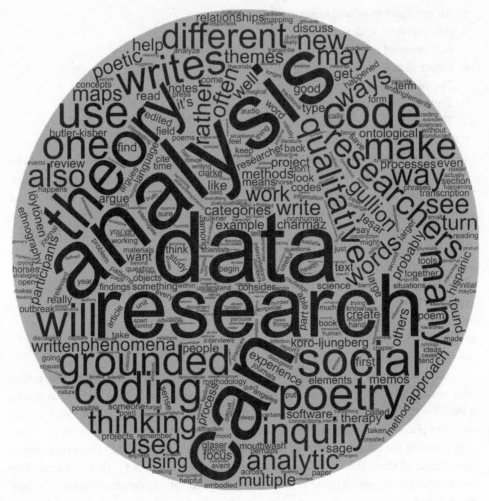

FIGURE 9.1 Word cloud.

be helpful to remember your initial research question: What is it that you wanted to know when you began this project? Focus on finding the answer. You may discover interesting patterns unrelated to your research question. Because we collect so much data for each project, we can usually write multiple articles (or a book) by approaching our data from different viewpoints. Thinking back to the horse therapy example—a paper could be written about how horse therapy is conducted. Another paper could be written on embodiment and therapy. Another could be on the meanings people attach to horse therapy (remember the magical code?).

It is likely that you've found all sorts of things you didn't expect—interesting things that have nothing to do with your research question. That's wonderful. Write your insights about that down and *come back to them later*. Qualitative data are so rich, if you've done your data collection well, you probably have lots of papers you could write (or a book or two) from your research. But we have to focus on one problem at a time. Use your research question to help guide your coding.

If you feel like you've tumbled into the Hell of Overcoding, step back from your data. If possible, don't look at your data for a few weeks. If you don't have that kind of time, at least do something to clear your head. Go for a walk or visit a museum or knit a scarf. Do whatever you like to do to relax. Then print an uncoded transcript and read it with your research question in mind. If you have a mentor or colleague who can look at your coding, that can also be helpful. They may be able to see connections you're overlooking.

There are a number of excellent software applications that can help you organize and code your data. Something as simple as a spreadsheet can be useful. I will not delve into software here. Software updates so frequently that I am concerned that whatever I write here would be out of date by the time you need them. Suffice to say that if you are coding a large data set, it would behoove you to learn how to use such applications. For smaller data sets, I personally find it easier to code by hand, using different colored markers or pens to mark different facets of the data set.

Categories

While we create analytic categories, we must also be mindful of their usefulness. Many social scientists rely on demographic variables, even when those data do not contribute to the analysis. Beck and Beck-Gernsheim (2002) call these zombie categories. They are zombies because they are dead—they don't help explain anything—yet we can't seem to bury them— we see them time and again in research. "Zombie categories are 'living dead' categories which govern our thinking but are not really able to capture the contemporary milieu" Beck and Beck-Gernsheim argue (cited in Slater and Ritzer 2001: 262), "What we really need is to redefine, reconstruct, restructure our concepts and our view of society."

Anytime we categorize people, we calcify the possibilities of their interactions. Social scientists love categories. Our favorites seem to be race and gender, but we also like to write about age and sexual proclivity and marital status. Researchers then compare people within the categories and look for differences and similarities. Hispanic babies have better outcomes than Black babies. Asians are more likely to have osteoporosis than other groups. Women live longer than men.

To be sure, categorization of people into different groups can provide us with fruitful information. Yet, these categories can also blind us to other possibilities. Jackson and Mazzei (2012: 10) invite us to interrogate this point. They ask, "Can there be useful knowledge if the traditional categories no longer hold?"

Demographics are helpful for comparing study to study; I don't argue that we should get rid of them. However, you should have a good answer for why you are using them in your study and ensure that you aren't using them for convenience sake. As an example, let's look at the variable Hispanic/non-Hispanic. This is a commonly used variable, a big tent that essentially means ancestry from the South of the United States. But Texas was part of Mexico, and many Texans have Indigenous ancestry. Are they Hispanic if they can trace their ancestry in Texas prior to it joining the United States? Or does that make them American? Does a person have to speak Spanish in order to be considered Hispanic? Or is Hispanic a proxy for "a brown person from the Americas"?

The term Hispanic erases many differences, including countries of origin. The lived experience of someone from Costa Rica is probably different from that of someone from Brazil (not to mention they probably don't speak the same primary language). With this being said, can we justifiably coalesce people into the broad category of Hispanic? Does that term tell us anything useful when researching health and illness? Maybe it does, but Hispanic is a broad category with great diversity of people who fall under that umbrella term. We are potentially missing a lot of information if we don't fine-tune our vision and explore multiple ways of knowing. Hispanic may be a category in your research, but how important is it to your research question? Are you using Hispanic when another variable might be more important?

As you code your data, interrogate why you code the way you do. Are you conforming to outdated traditions? Or are you thinking about your data in new and innovative ways? Are you repeating settler–colonialist perspectives, or can you decolonize your thinking?

Grounded Theory

The bulk of this section is based on the work of Kathy Charmaz (2014), who is broadly considered one of the key figures in the field of grounded theory methodology, just as Saldaña is considered a key figure in coding. Charmaz builds off the pivotal foundation of Barney Glaser and Anselm Strauss (both of whom she studied with in graduate school). Glaser and Strauss are credited with the development of grounded theory, with their publication of *The Discovery of Grounded Theory: Strategies for Qualitative Research*, in 1967.

Qualitative scholars use grounded theory for theory construction itself. That is, rather than having a theoretical underpinning to their research, the problem they are working on needs its own theory. Charmaz (2014: 1) writes that

> researchers construct a theory "grounded" in their data. Grounded theory begins with inductive data, invokes iterative strategies of going back and forth between data and analysis, uses comparative methods, and keeps you interacting and involved with your data and emerging analysis.

This is a well-developed, systematic process. Although we discuss it here, scholars truly wishing to do this type of theory construction are urged to read Charmaz and other authors who write about theory construction in depth before calling their work "grounded theory." As you will see, many of the techniques we review in this chapter overlap within and between methods. Be clear about which technique you are using and why you are using it. Some researchers will call their work grounded theory when they have not engaged in theory construction (save yourself that embarrassment and get this correct).

Although grounded theory techniques are evolving, they are based on positivism, influenced by the science of quantitative methods, and tend to embrace many of the same assumptions ontologically and epistemologically. Charmaz (2014: 9) writes that "[Glaser] imbued the methods with dispassionate empiricism, rigorous codified methods, emphasis on emergent discoveries, and its somewhat ambiguous specialized language that echoes quantitative methods." This makes sense when we consider that Glaser and Strass' book was written in the late 1960s, when the social sciences were fighting to be recognized in the academy as "serious" and losing funding to the laboratory sciences, which were considered to be more rigorous. Given its American roots, it's also not surprising that grounded theory also has pragmatic undertones. Although grounded theory is not as rigid today as in its roots (indeed, Glaser and Strass parted ways on this point), it is nonetheless a rigorous means for data analysis (Charmaz 2014).

Grounded theory is a means for theory construction, but the theories that emerge are seldom universal and more of what sociologists refer to as "theories of the middle range" (Merton 1949). Theories generated from grounded analysis are specific to well-defined cases (Charmaz 2014: 10).

When beginning grounded theory research, many authors advise that you not begin with a literature review but instead go into the field "cold." This way, they argue, you will be less influenced by what others have discovered. Of course, it is impossible not to be influenced by our pre-existing knowledges and standpoints, so I'm not sure how valuable this advice is. As we discussed with reflexivity, interrogate your preconceptions both before you enter the field and while you are doing your research. Charmaz, Thornberg, and Keane (2018: 419), express concern that in not engaging prior research, a grounded theorist could wind up with a "trivial product" without the nuances that prior research could have afforded.

Charmaz (2010: 11) writes that grounded theorists

1. Conduct data collection and analysis simultaneously in an iterative process
2. Analyze actions and processes rather than themes and structure
3. Use comparative methods
4. Draw on data (e.g., narratives and descriptions) in service of developing new conceptual categories
5. Develop inductive analytical categories through systematic data analysis
6. Emphasize theory construction rather than description or application of current theories
7. Engage in theoretical sampling
8. Search for variation in the studied categories or process
9. Pursue developing a category rather than covering a specific empirical topic.

Analysis is an iterative process. Grounded theorists make many passes through their data, using many different types of coding strategies. They do this to identify analytic categories and to discover connections between them. While working with their data, grounded theorists write analytic memos. These are similar to memos that ethnographers write in the field—thoughts about what they see happening in the data.

Charmaz (2014) recommends that researchers begin by reading through their transcriptions and make a pass at what she calls initial coding. In this type of coding, you want to look at words and brief phrases and code them, often with the words the participants actually use. This is different from using a theory to guide your coding. If we were coding to reconstruct a theory, or to think with a theory, we would use the theory to guide our coding instead.

In the initial phase, you look at small fragments of data. This is followed by what Charmaz (2014) calls focused coding, during which the researcher considers larger batches of text. At this stage, Charmaz (2014: 113) writes that we "[use] the most significant or frequent initial codes to sort, synthesize, integrate, and organize large amounts of data." Once we coalesce our codes into categories, we look for relationships between categories. We then construct an analytic model (a theory).

Situational Analysis and Data Mapping

In 2005, Adele E. Clarke published her book, *Situational Analysis: Grounded Theory After the Postmodern Turn*. Most of this section is derived from that text. Clarke is a colleague of Charmaz and student of Strauss, and she extends their work through a postmodern framing.

Clarke (2005: xxii; bold and italics in original) introduces three "cartographic approaches" to data analysis:

1. **Situational maps** that lay out the major human, nonhuman, discursive, and other elements in the research situation of inquiry and provoke analysis of relations among them;
2. **Social worlds/arenas maps** that lay out the collective actors, nonhuman elements, and the arena(s) of commitment and discourse within which they are engaged in ongoing negotiations—meso-level interpretations of the situations; and
3. **Positional maps** that lay out the major positions taken, and *not* taken, in the data vis-à-vis particular axes of difference, concern, and controversy around issues in the situation of inquiry.

Clarke (2005) designed her techniques to shift the focus of grounded theory away from individuals as the unit of analysis to phenomena or situations as the unit of analysis. Social scientists are often interested in phenomena rather than in individuals; however, because of limitations in our ability to sample phenomena, we tend to sample people and then use that data to understand phenomena. Clarke's technique allows us to sample phenomena instead.

Situatedness in the postmodern turn, according to Clarke (2005), involves recognition that our means of inquiry often smooth over the complexity of human social life. She writes that

> methods are needed that can address and elucidate the complexities of situations as the grounds of social life . . . that intentionally aim at capturing complexities rather than aiming at simplifications; that elucidate processes of change in situations as well as they educate patterns and stabilities; that detangle agents and positions sufficiently to make contradictions, ambivalences, and irrelevances clear. (p. xxix)

As such, she invites us to include objects, discourses, and structures at different "levels" (micro, mezzo, macro) in our analyses.

Situational analysis or data mapping is particularly useful for people who enjoy thinking visually. To begin mapping the data, look at the codes that you have used. What is important in this situation? Clarke (2005) recommends you write this out on a large sheet of paper (you could do this digitally or with concept mapping software as well). This allows you to literally see what is happening in your research.

Clarke (2005) recommends you photocopy the maps you create so that you can write and/or draw on them or arrange the elements in different ways. Be sure to save all of the copies you work on. The same applies to digital versions. Save each with a new name. Review the copies, go back to old versions, ensure that you didn't delete anything or miss any connections. This is good advice to follow throughout your research project. Save everything. If you want to delete parts of your writing, save it in a separate document. You never know when you will want to go back and retrieve something.

Once you've made your initial maps, you can begin revising them. Clarke (2005: 89) writes that "simply staring at the situational map, revising it via collapsing and expanding categories/items, adding and deleting, is analytically productive."

The next step in Clark's (2005) mapping process is to begin what she calls relational analysis. That is, you want to consider the relationships between and among the elements on your maps. As before, you can do this by hand or digitally, and you should keep each version. Through many iterations, Clarke (2005: 102) asks us to look at every interaction between and among every possible connection on our map. As you consider those relationships, memo about them.

Similar to concept maps, Butler-Kisber (2010) writes about the use of collage as both a data collection technique (through collage elicitation) and a tool for analysis to see the webs of connection present in the data. She writes, "Collage evokes embodied responses, and uses juxtaposition of fragments and the presence of ambiguity to engage the viewer in multiple avenues of interpretation" (p. 103). Collage helps give light to unconscious ideas about the project, and it is one means of contemplative practice. Rather than provide us with certainty, collage introduces uncertainty, allowing the researcher to express emotions about the project in ways that are sensory and embodied. Butler-Kisber writes that "the creator seeks the fragments and glues them together to express a feeling or sense of an experience of phenomenon rather than a particular idea" (p. 104).

This is similar to poetry as method, as we will see. Butler-Kisber writes, "A collage starts from the feeling. Each collage . . . reveals a certain intuitive facet of the question/phenomenon that emerges when trying to portray a feeling in response to the research question" (p. 116). Maps and collages may be used to help understand a problem and write up one's findings.

Poetic Inquiry

Toxic Neighborhood

The ground trembles beneath my bare feet. Truck after truck rumbles up my street, hauling crack/frack fluid (water, chemicals) to the natural gas drilling site at the end of my block.

Injecting their fluid into the earth.

Penetrating, cracking her open.

She rumbles.

We've had three earthquakes in so many days. A man in a gray suit comes on TV. He says the earthquakes aren't related to the drilling. (Never mind we never had quakes here before).

I live in the middle of the Barnett Shale, in a suburban town not far from Dallas. Tucked in my neighborhood are natural gas pads. Pipelines crisscross behind our fences. There are more than three hundred sites in town.

Air alert! It's a Red Day. The children cannot play outside; the air is dangerous to breathe. They ask to go swimming—Mama, it's summer, it's hot out. No, I tell them, let's go after dinner when there is shade. I don't tell them breathing outside is deadly (I don't want to frighten them).

The drill towers about a hundred feet above our homes. They call it a Christmas tree, but there's nothing festive about it.

Jenny, the woman across the street, found a lump in her breast. She has stage three breast cancer. Jenny is 29.

Elizabeth lives two houses down. Her daughter has leukemia and has no hair. The PTA had a fund-raiser to help them pay for chemo. Then Charlie's daughter was diagnosed. And then Tori's son.

Our spare change won't go that far.

So many of our neighbors have cancer that the school district started a support group. It meets at our elementary school.

The Texas Department of State Health Services says we are a statistical anomaly, not a cancer cluster.

Nothing to see here, folks. Move along.

Some of our neighbors tried to organize against the gas companies. We don't care that they drill here, we said, but we want them to be safe about it. There is an activist who comes to our meetings with a dummy dressed in overalls and a gas mask. She calls him Ben Zene, because benzene is always at the gas sites and she doesn't want anyone to forget. You learn all about these chemicals and how they cause cancer when these things come into your neighborhood. It's like being Erin Brockovich.

We protested at the site. We wore paper gas masks and put paper gas masks on our children. We had signs—Get the Frack Out of Our Town! and Fracking Pollutes! and Our Children Can't Breathe! We tied the signs to the fence. The next day we found our signs vandalized with drawings of genitalia.

Pussy, one said.

You're next.

We watch the commercials, a man in pressed jeans, cowboy boots. He's someone famous. He stands in a lush pasture, show horses graze in the background. He tells us natural gas will bring jobs and that it is a greener alternative. The camera zooms in on the top of a drill. Someone has attached an American flag, it flutters in the breeze. Natural gas will free us from dependence on foreign oil, the nice-looking man says. We will finally be free.

My cousin berates me for being unpatriotic when I complain. Give me a break, he says, where do you think electricity comes from? He throws up his hands in disgust.

I feel small.

I just want them to do it safely, I whisper.

I don't want my kids to get cancer.

There's this blogger I read. She lives just a few miles from my house, in a neighboring town. She started seeing weird stuff in her yard, what looked like bubbling frack fluid, in her yard. She's on well water and she had her water tested. It was contaminated with all sorts of chemicals.

She tried to light her water on fire, like they do in that documentary, *Gasland*. She videotaped it and put it on her blog. She filled the basin and tried to light it. The water didn't catch fire, but after she'd held the flame to the water, she swished her hand around in it. When she pulled her hand out, there was a film hanging from it, it looked just like Saran Wrap.

That's petrochemicals. If you can make plastic with flame, you have petrochemicals in your water.

The blogger tried to sell her house, but after the wells went in her property value dropped by seventy-five percent. No one will buy these houses. We are trapped.

I call the city: We can't help you.

I call the health department: We can't help you.

I call the Texas Commission on Environmental Quality: We can't help you.

I call the Railroad Commission: We can't help you.

I call the Environmental Protection Agency: We can't help you.

I call my Senator: We can't help you.

I am surrounded by a lack of competent guardians.

I put down the phone.

Grass fires burn along the freeway. Fields of corn crumble to dust. My flowerbed withers and browns. We are under Stage Four Drought Rationing. We cannot water the lawns.

Meanwhile five million gallons of water are diverted to crack/frack the well up the block. Five million gallons lost, contaminated with chemicals and radiation. Any water that flows back up to the surface will be hauled back out by those trucks to an empty well and injected thousands of feet below ground, lost to our generation and generations to come.

The ground trembles beneath my bare feet. Truck after truck rumbles up my street, hauling crack/frack fluid (water, chemicals) to the natural gas drilling site at the end of my block. I wipe my nose with the back of my hand. It is bleeding again.

—Gullion (2013: ix–xi)

The above poem incorporates field notes, in-depth interview transcripts, and creative non-fiction to create a composite character that reflects the impact of fracking in a neighborhood. My goal was not only to show what it is like for residents who live next to fracking sites but also to portray some of their emotional responses, feelings of helplessness, and the gut punch of the failure of the regulatory agencies to help.

> Poetic inquiry involves the use of poetry as an interrogative device.

In this section, I draw from Sandra Faulker's work on poetic inquiry. Poetic inquiry involves the use of poetry as an interrogative device at different stages of a project. It can be used as a form of analysis and of representation. Faulkner (2020: 14) writes,

> "Poetic inquiry" is the use of poetry crafted from research endeavors, either before project analysis, as a project analysis, and/or poetry that is part of or that constitutes an entire research project. The key feature of poetic inquiry is the use of poetry as/in/for inquiry.

Poetic inquiry invites us to explore the emotions and emotional responses entangled in our research. It also forces us to consider our use of language. Sometimes a written report doesn't get at the marrow of what a researcher is trying to express. Poetry can help evoke affective responses in readers that you may be unable to portray in traditional research reports. There is a focus on the aesthetics of our prose and the lyrical qualities of our writing. There is an embodied quality to poetry: "Feminist scholars, women of color, and practitioners have been interested in embodiment, experimental knowledge and theories of the flesh for quite some time," Faulkner (2020: 19) writes. Poetry has long been used as a means to evoke affective responses in the reader. It can help a reader feel whatever the researcher is trying to express, in radical empathy.

Poetry can also be a tool for anti-colonial and anti-racist projects. Faulkner (2020: 21) writes that

> ethnopoetics pay careful attention to language in an attempt to decrease distance between researchers and those being researched, between mind and body, and to critique colonization and representations of non-Western cultures through a focus on aesthetic differences between Western literary traditions and indigenous orality.

One type of poetic inquiry is found poetry. In making a found poem, the researcher extracts words and phrases from a document (often an interview transcript) and makes them into a poetic form. Butler-Kisber (2010: 84) writes, "Found poetry is the rearrangement of words, phrases, and sometimes whole passages that are taken from other sources and reframed as poetry by changes in spacing and/or lines (and consequently meaning), or by altering the text by additions and/or deletions." Butler-Kisber notes that "poetry hides . . . in the transcript" (p. 87). Our job is to find the poems.

Poems can be written from all sorts of data and at different times in your research process. Aside from finding poems in interview transcripts, you can also write poems based on your observations or cobble them together from your field notes, memos, or research journals. Blackout poetry is made when someone has a page of text and then removes words, leaving behind words that make up a poem. You can also make poems from your codes.

Some journals don't publish poetry or poetic analysis, so before you send an article off only to be rejected, make sure the journal will accept it. Conversely, there are many peer-reviewed poetry journals that you might wish to consider. Many poets also self-publish or work with small independent presses to publish chapbooks. A chapbook is a collection of poems around one theme.

Faulkner (2020: 4) writes,

> I write poetry because I am a bad (BAD!) social scientist. I study personal relationships; I am most interested in what relationships feel like and sound like and smell like more than how they function as some kind of analytic variable to be deconstructed. I believe in poetic truth(s) more than social science Truth punctuated with a capital T. . . . What I understand is that one can write poetry as social science.

Analyzing your data with different forms of representation can be a method for thinking deeply with them (Weaver-Hightower 2019). For example, you can code the data and write poetry with them, or you can create concept maps and write an ethnodrama. There are multiple ways to engage with your data, to think deeply about your research.

Post-Qualitative Inquiry

Now that I've spent many pages telling you about coding, I confess that I don't code my data. I used to, and I have reams of coded data from previous projects. Coding is a useful way to analyze your data, but it is not the only way.

Jackson and Mazzei (2012) propose that we not code data. They argue that coding pushes the researcher away from the data—that it collapses rich information down and minimizes it. They worry that coding data serves as a technique to scientificize what we already knew before we conducted the study. Instead, they argue for working with a theoretical concept (e.g., Foucault's notion of power or Butler's performativity) and then work through the data with that concept, noting both how the concept informs the data and how the data inform the concept.

Jackson and Mazzei (2012) also push back against the practice of *creating* themes/categories/variables as a way to open possibilities for insight. Instead, they argue, in a Deleuzian fashion, for deterritorializing of empirical material. This is a radical shift from traditional, humanist qualitative research. To do this type of analysis, they argue for "plugging" one text in/through another. They "read" data through theory. They deconstruct themes/categories/variables in interesting ways. This goes beyond using a theory to help create and understand your project, instead calls for using data in deep intra-action with the theoretical concepts under deterritorialization. They use that intra-action to push the boundaries of what the theory can know.

The end product of our coding or other data analysis technique is a co-constructed reality. Analysis will always be through the lens of the researcher, and we cannot escape the fact that our interpretations of the empirical materials we collected might differ from those of the participants. This is not simply a matter for qualitative researchers to consider. Quantitative researchers also distill human experience.

A current debate among qualitative methodologists has to do with traditional humanist qualitative research (which most of this book deals with) and post-qualitative inquiry. I include this section because this debate is such a prominent schism in the academic community. We begin with a discussion of "data."

Denzin (2017) writes that using the term data invites criticisms of validity, reliability, and objectivity, that might not be relevant to the type of method a researcher is using. The term invokes positivism, which is fine when one approaches research from a positivist orientation but is incorrect when researching through other philosophical lenses. Koro-Ljungberg, Löytönen, and Tesar (2017: 2) write that "the term data has been argued to carry an odour of scientificity, lending a spurious scientific rigor to the critical and cultural projects of qualitative research, alongside such concepts as validity and triangulation."

Post-qualitative researchers "interrogate the practices and politics of evidence that produce data. They support the call for new ways of making the mundane, taken for granted everyday world visible" (Denzin 2017: 82).

We thus return to the question of science and the roots of social science inquiry. Is what we are doing "scientific"? Does it have to be in order to be worthwhile? One can understand the benefits being labeled scientific within the academy: Science garners more prestige (and, by association, more funding) than the arts and humanities. Yet as we peel back the layers of scientificity, we find the assumptions that are made about science, about how one does science, to be problematic (Gullion 2018). As Duhn (2017: 13) writes, "The modernist dream of clean, objective, pure data that reveals the concrete truth about reality and enables the making of better futures, is an illusion."

There are many valid ways of knowing a thing, and being open to different ways of knowing gives us different perspectives on the thing. "Rather than collecting or even producing data," Koro-Ljungberg et al. (2017: 1) write, "we focus on data encounters and diverse ways in which scholars and data (in their multiple forms) can come together, interact, intra-act, and."

In her keynote address at the 2013 International Congress of Qualitative Inquiry, Elizabeth St. Pierre (2013) argued that methodology is an "apparatus of capture." More than once I have heard her discuss the fact that qualitative methods (any methods, really) were something we invented. Post-qualitative researchers are concerned about the reification of method. Methods are tools that people created for particular situations. Sometimes we may need to make up new tools, and that is a good thing. Post-qualitative researchers call for fluidity. They argue that we stop the movement when we call something data, pin it down like a butterfly, encase it in amber, destroying the agential capacity of data.

Kuntz (2019) argues that our inquiry should be philosophical in nature (this is similar, but not quite the same, as Jackson and Mazzei's [2012] notion of thinking with theory). Like other post-qualitative thinkers engaging the ontological turn, Kunze argues our focus should be on what events happen and how they work, rather on why people do what they do. He writes,

> All too often, discussions of *why* slip into a type of simplistic socio-psychological analysis that fails the project at hand. Often, this failure extends from a cultural fixation on first (or primary) causes that lead to a cascading array of effects. In this scenario, the only way to instigate significant change is to, in some way, challenge the replication of that cause (or to show it as unjust in some way). Quite simply, I do not recognize that approach as useful for any type of legitimate social change. It is a fool's errand. (p. 3)

This is a switch from focusing on meaning and meaning-making activities (epistemology) to the nature of reality (ontology). Post-qualitative researchers strive to open potential avenues for understanding, rather than replicating what we already know. The takeaway point here is that it is ok for your research process to be messy. It is ok to make up new techniques for doing research if your project calls for it. Nothing I've written about in this book should be taken as gospel.

We've discussed a number of different ways to analyze your data. The foundation of each is that they are a way to help you *organize* and *think* about your data. Qualitative projects amass a lot of empirical materials. It can be difficult to put all the pieces together and understand what is happening at a deep level theoretically. Thinking is hard. There is no straightforward answer. We do not solve for *x*. Weaver-Hightower (2019: 14) addresses this beautifully:

> As I look across the analytical process that led to "Waltzing Matilda" [his autoethnography about his stillborn daughter], the distributed, wild, and hybrid nature of my analysis fascinates me. Analysis happened informally as well as formally. It happened simultaneously with collecting artifacts and living experiences. Analysis happened within my lifeworld and in reading about others' lifeworlds. It happened of my own volition, through dialogue with others, as a reaction to peer review. Analysis happened in pictures and prose, before writing as well as during and after.

References

Beck, Ulrich, and Elizabeth Beck-Gernsheim. 2002. *Individualization: Institutional Individualism and Its Social and Political Consequences*. Thousand Oaks, CA: SAGE.

Butler-Kisber, Lynn. 2010. *Qualitative Inquiry: Thematic, Narrative and Arts-Informed Perspectives*. Los Angeles: SAGE.

Charmaz, Kathy. 2010. "Studying the Experience of Chronic Illness Through Grounded Theory." In *New Directions in the Sociology of Chronic and Disabling Conditions: Assaults on the Lifeworld*, edited by Graham Scambler and Sasha Scambler, 8–36. London: Palgrave.

Charmaz, Kathy. 2014. *Constructing Grounded Theory*, 2nd ed. Los Angeles: SAGE.

Charmaz, Kathy, Robert Thornberg, and Elaine Keane. 2018. "Evolving Grounded Theory and Social Justice Inquiry." In *The SAGE handbook of qualitative research*, edited by Norman K. Denzin and Yvonna S. Lincoln, 411–443. Thousand Oaks, CA: SAGE.

Clarke, Adele E. 2005. *Situational Analysis: Grounded Theory After the Postmodern Turn*. Los Angeles: SAGE.

Denzin, Norman K. 2017. "Data: The Wonder of It All." In *Disrupting Data in Qualitative Inquiry: Entanglements with the Post-Critical and Post-Anthropocentric*, edited by Mirka Koro-Ljungberg, Teija Löytönen, and Marek Tesar, 81–91. New York: Lang.

Duhn, Iris. 2017. "Performing Data." In *Disrupting Data in Qualitative Inquiry: Entanglements with the Post-Critical and Post-Anthropocentric*, edited by Mirka Koro-Ljungberg, Teija Löytönen, and Marek Tesar, 11–21. New York: Lang.

Faulkner, Sandra L. 2020. *Poetic Inquiry: Craft, Method and Practice*, 2nd ed. London: Routledge.

Glaser, Barney G., and Anselm L. Strauss. 1967. *The Discovery of Grounded Theory: Strategies for Qualitative Research*. Chicago: Aldine.

Gullion, Jessica Smartt. 2013. "Toxic Neighborhood." *Qualitative Inquiry* 19, no. 7: 491–492.

Gullion, Jessica Smartt. 2015. *Fracking the Neighborhood: Reluctant Activists and Natural Gas Drilling*. Cambridge, MA: MIT Press.

Gullion, Jessica Smartt. 2018. *Diffractive Ethnography: Social Sciences in the Ontological Turn*. London: Routledge.

Humble, Áine M., and M. Elise Radina. 2019. *How Qualitative Data Analysis Happens: Moving Beyond "Themes Emerged."* London: Routledge.

Jackson, Alecia Y., and Lisa A. Mazzei. 2012. *Thinking with Theory in Qualitative Research: Viewing Data Across Multiple Perspectives*. New York: Routledge.

Koro-Ljungberg, Mirka, Teija Löytönen, and Marek Tesar. 2017. "Introduction: Multiplicities of Data Encounters." In *Disrupting Data in Qualitative Inquiry: Entanglements with the Post-Critical and Post-Anthropocentric*, edited by Mirka Koro-Ljungberg, Teija Löytönen, and Marek Tesar, 1–9. New York: Lang.

Kuntz, Aaron M. 2019. *Qualitative Inquiry, Cartography, and the Promise of Material Change*. London: Routledge.

Merton, Robert K. 1949. *Social Theory and Social Structure*. New York: Simon & Schuster.

Rosenblatt, Paul C., and Elizabeth Wieling. 2019. "Thematic and Phenomenological Analysis in Research on Intimate Relationships." In *How Qualitative Data Analysis Happens: Moving Beyond "Themes Emerged,"* edited by Áine H. Humble and M. Elise Radina, 50–63. London: Routledge.

Saldaña, Johnny. 2011. *Fundamentals of Qualitative Research*. New York: Oxford University Press.

Saldaña, Jonny. 2016. *The Coding Manual for Qualitative Researchers*, 3rd ed. Los Angeles: SAGE.

Slater, John, and George Ritzer. (2001). "Interview with Urich Beck." *Journal of Consumer Culture* 1, no. 2: 261–277.

St. Pierre, Elizabeth Adams. 2013. "The Appearance of Data." *Cultural Studies ↔ Critical Methodologies* 13, no. 4: 223–227.

Weaver-Hightower, Marcus B. 2019. "Analyzing Self and Other in Autoethnography," In *How Qualitative Data Analysis Happens: Moving Beyond "Themes Emerged,"* edited by Áine H. Humble and M. Elise Radina, 3–17. London: Routledge.

FURTHER READING

Alexander, Bryant Keith, and Mary E. Weems. 2022. *Collaborative Spirit-Writing and Performance in Everyday Black Lives*. New York: Routledge.

Lather, Patti. 2017. *(Post)Critical Methodologies: The Science Possible After the Critiques, the Selected Works of Patti Lather*. New York: Routledge.

Discussion Questions

1. What is coding? Why might a researcher want to code their data?
2. How might someone use poetic inquiry in their research?

Active Learning

1. Give each member of the class the same set of data. The biblical chapter Leviticus is good for this exercise. Have them code the data individually. Then put them in pairs to see how similarly or differently they coded the data. Have them code the data again together and then draw conclusions about what they found in the data.
2. Create a found poem from an interview transcript that captures the emotional essence of the participant's words.

Mindfulness Exercises

1. Think about your own critical thinking skills. Map out how you go about thinking deeply about a problem or issue.
2. Does poetry resonate with you? Can poetry be social science?

10

Reporting Results

Given the nature of health research, reporting results could take a variety of forms. In this chapter, we explore how to write up results for a variety of audiences. We begin with a discussion of writing for traditional peer-reviewed journals and examine both conventional and nonconventional writing styles. This is followed by a discussion of voice and who is allowed to speak for another person. We then transition into general mechanics of writing well and how to edit your work.

The final step in any research project is to share the results with the scholarly community. We do this through publication. Richardson (2009: 308) writes,

> Unlike quantitative work which can carry its meaning in its tables and summaries, qualitative work carries its meanings in its entire text. Just as a piece of literature is not equivalent to its "plot summary," qualitative research is not contained in its abstract. Qualitative research has to be read, not scanned; its meaning is in the reading.

Qualitative research provides us with comprehensive data to draw from. Learning to write well helps ensure that our research is read and that readers are able to understand the meaning in the reading.

"All scientific writing is storytelling," Denzin (2010: 92) reminds us. Even when we give our audience a dry piece of prose, we are trying to convince them we are correct, that our findings matter, and that our findings should matter to them. Our writing tells the story of our research.

Peer-Reviewed Publications

We begin with a discussion of how to write for peer-reviewed journals, because most academics must have this sort of publication in order to be considered for promotion and

Qualitative Research in Health and Illness. Jessica Smartt Gullion, Oxford University Press. © Oxford University Press 2024.
DOI: 10.1093/oso/9780190915988.003.0011

tenure. Increasingly, search committees expect to see that PhD candidates in the job market also have multiple peer-reviewed journal publications listed on their vitas.

Before submitting your work to a journal, take the time to understand what type of work that journal publishes, and determine whether your work "fits" with that type. For example, if you are writing about the emergency room care experiences of women who have been raped, you should search for medical and nursing journals that will be open to the topic. If you are writing about body image, you might look to gender studies or psychology journals. Make sure that the topic of your article fits within the editorial scope of the journal. If not, the article won't be published, and you will have wasted both your time and that of the editor.

One way to identify possible journals to submit your work to is to look at the reference list of the article you are writing. In which journals were those articles published? Those journals may be more open to publishing your piece.

Nearly all journals have websites on which you should be able to find information about their editorial vision. You should also be able to find tables of contents for the most recent issues. Look through them. Does your article seem to fit within their scope? If all of the articles are quantitative, search for a different journal. Even if the topic of your piece fits the mission of the journal, it is unlikely that it will publish qualitative research. When you find a journal that seems to be a good fit, pull some of the most recent articles to see how they were formatted. Did they have long literature reviews? Did any of them mention reflexivity? How much space was devoted to data analysis methods? This will help you tailor your paper to that journal.

One you decide on a particular journal, read the guidelines for authors. Generally, these guidelines will provide information about how to format your submission. Follow those closely; many articles are rejected for simply not following these guidelines.

To submit your paper for consideration, you will likely be asked to upload it to the journal's website. There, you will also be invited to write a letter to the editors. This is your chance to briefly sell your piece. Tell them what the paper is about, why it fits the scope of their journal, and why you are the right person to have written this article. This does not need to be lengthy; a few sentences will do.

Once your paper has been submitted, it will be reviewed by an editor at the journal for fit. At this point, your paper may be "desk rejected" and not sent out for review. This usually happens if your work diverges too far from what the journal publishes, is too similar to something they just published, or it has too many glaring errors (including that you didn't follow the guidelines for authors). As an example, there is a qualitative health journal that refuses to publish poetic analysis. It states this on its website. If you send it poetry, the journal will reject it, even if the paper is well written. It's simply outside of the scope of the journal. If you are desk rejected, it is seldom worth your time and energy to argue with the editor; find another journal to submit your work to.

If the editor decides your paper has merit, they will send it out for peer review. Usually, between two and four scholars will blind review the paper. They will not know any identifying information about you personally. They will offer feedback on the paper based on a rubric the journal has created for this purpose.

The peer-review process is often time-consuming. Sometimes the journal editors will have difficulty finding people willing to review. They may have difficulty finding people to review who have the proper expertise for your paper. Sometimes people agree to conduct a review and then forget about doing it. All sorts of things can hold up the process, and unfortunately, you just have to be patient. If you have not heard back after six months, send a kind inquiry to the editor as to the status of your paper. Know, however, that papers can take a year or two to move through the system.

As a side note, this is why we should review papers for journals when invited, and to review them in a timely manner. The system does not work if we are not willing to play our part. It is also good practice for us as researchers to be ready to write the next article while the first one is being reviewed (this is called "having something in the pipeline," and you always want to have something in the pipeline to keep your research trajectory moving forward).

Once your paper has been reviewed, you will receive one of the following outcomes: reject, revise and resubmit, accept with minor revisions, or outright accept. Most papers are either rejected or receive an invitation to revise and resubmit. If you are asked to revise the paper, the editor will provide you with a list of items to revise. If you want the journal to publish your paper, you must address all of the items.

This doesn't mean you can't push back against editors' requests. If they are asking something that is impossible, tell them so. Perhaps they want a revision with data you did not collect, or they want you to change the research design. It's ok to explain why you cannot take some of their suggestions, but know that also means your paper may not end up being published.

I once went through three rounds of revise and resubmit with a journal. The reviewers wanted data I didn't collect, they wanted me to follow up on an incidental finding and make it the focus of the paper, and they wanted me to use a completely different theoretical lens to my project. In the end, I decided not to publish with that journal and found a different outlet.

> Journal publishing is a finicky business. Never take rejection personally.

Journal publishing is a finicky business. Never take rejection personally. Rejection simply means that *this* journal is not interested in *this* particular piece of writing. It does not mean that you are a poor scholar or that your ideas don't have value. Thousands of legitimate journals exist. If your paper is rejected, use any helpful feedback that may have been given, and then send your work someplace else.

I have two more pieces of advice about journal publishing. The first pertains to predatory journals, and the second has to do with journal impact factors.

Predatory journals are in the business of making money off of academics. The owners understand how important publishing is to our careers, and they take advantage of that. These journals may also be known as "pay to play" outlets. The author pays a fee (usually in the thousands of dollars), and the article is published.

Because thousands of journals exist, sometimes it can be difficult to determine if a journal you are considering is legitimate or not. This is made more problematic by the increase in open access resources, which also require the author to pay exorbitant fees. If you are unsure about the validity of any journal, your university library should be able to assist you. There are also many lists of predatory journals on the internet. You do not want one of these on your vita; it will damage your credibility as a scholar.

On the other side of the spectrum, the top journals have high-impact factors. The impact factor can usually be found on the journal's website. This is a measure of how often articles in that journal (on average) are cited by other authors. "High" is relative to the discipline, however. For example, the *Journal of the American Medical Association* has an impact factor of 56.272. The *American Sociological Review* has an impact factor of 9.654. Both of these journals are flagship journals in their respective fields. The more niche the field you are working in, the lower the impact factor will probably be, even for the most respected journals in that field.

Some universities, particularly research intensive (R1 universities in the United States), expect their faculty to publish in high-impact journals. Other universities may care less about this as long as the journal is legitimate and the article is peer-reviewed. Find out what the expectation is at your university.

Writing a Traditional-Style Research Paper

Although there are many ways to write up the results of your research, we begin by discussing the traditional-style research paper. Scientific papers have the same basic structure. If you deconstruct the articles in most scientific or positivist journals, regardless of discipline, you will see the following sections, in this order:

- Introduction
- Review of the literature
- Theoretical framework
- Method
- Data
- Findings
- Discussion
- Conclusion

Using this outline, the author plugs in relevant information into relevant sections.

The introduction does what it says it does. It introduces the reader to what to expect from the rest of the paper. The introduction is brief—at most three or four paragraphs—and ends with the research question that guides the project.

Next, the author reviews literature relevant to the research study. All of the previous research that has been conducted on the particular research question should be reviewed. In this way, the author's research is contextualized within the larger body of research.

Alongside the review of the literature is a discussion of the theoretical framework that informed the research. The writer should show how that framework has been used to study similar research questions.

In the method section, the author explains how they collected and analyzed the data for the study. There should be mention of Institutional Review Board (IRB) approval (if human subjects were involved) in this section as well. The author should demonstrate why *this* method was the best way to respond to *this* research question. The author will then discuss the data that they collected. Usually they begin with an overview of the data set—for example, discussing the *N*-size and demographics. This gives the reader a sense of the quality and quantity of the data collected.

In the findings section, the researcher writes in-depth about what they discovered after data analysis. They will often use quotes or other examples from the data to support their claims.

In the discussion section, the findings are tied back to the literature review and theory. How did this study further the scholarly conversation about this topic? Was something new discovered? Did it expand what we know in some way? Was anything counter to the previous literature on this topic?

Finally, the article ends with a one or two paragraph conclusion. This generally includes a summary of the major implications of the research, acknowledgment of any limitations of the research, and suggestions for further research on the topic.

This paper structure is very common in health journals, and it should be easy to discern when you are reviewing literature. Although formulaic, there is nothing to stop the writer from making the paper an interesting read. Formulaic does not have to be boring.

Writing a Nontraditional Research Paper

There are all sorts of other ways to write peer-reviewed papers that do not follow the above structure. Just as qualitative research is open to alternative ways of knowing, the field also is much more open to alternative ways of writing. Check the journal you are considering to determine how much variety they print.

There are journals for creative nonfiction, social fiction, poetry, autoethnography, ethnodrama, photo essays, and so on. Peer-reviewed doesn't mean stodgy. It means that peers in your field—subject matter experts—have read your work and believe that it is worthy of publication.

You can represent your findings in many different ways. A particular research study might warrant a traditional peer-reviewed journal article and an art installation, for example. The two different mediums allow for different points of entry and connection to your research. They also invite different audiences to engage with the work.

When using any arts-based research practice, the

Arts-based researchers use a variety of artistic forms to understand their data and to represent their findings.

researcher must be well-versed in qualitative methods as well as the artistic medium they choose to employ. This doesn't mean you have to be the best painter, poet, or novelist, but it does mean that you work on your craft as much as the other components of the project. This is one difficulty of any arts-based research project. You need to produce both good social science and good art.

As an example, Faulkner (2020: 144) offers a schema for evaluating poetic inquiry, both scientific and artistic. Scientific criteria include depth, authenticity, trustworthiness, understanding of human experience, reflexivity, usefulness, articulation of method, and ethical considerations. Likewise, Faulker argues, there are artistic criteria, including compression of data, understanding of craft, social justice, moral truth, emotional verisimilitude, evocation, sublime, and empathy. To evaluate poetic inquiry (and I argue the same for any other form of arts-based research), we look at where the two realms—science and art—overlap. Faulkner argues these include artistic concentration, embodied experience, discovery/surprise, conditionality, narrative truth, and transformation.

Leavy (2020) argues for something similar but also recognizes that the art does not have to be best to get the point across. You must still attend to the crafting of the piece. If you are not doing good art, you risk losing your audience.

No matter how you present your results, maintain transparency with your reader. Tell the reader what you are doing and why. If you are fictionalizing stories from your research to protect identities, let the reader know. If you are making found poems from interview transcripts, explain your process. Even if you write in a scientific style, explain to your reader what you did. This transparency lends credibility to your choices.

Writing for Other Publications

Peer-reviewed journal articles tend to be inaccessible to lay readers. If a reader is not affiliated with a university or doesn't have access to another subscription clearinghouse, they will find that many journal articles are protected by firewalls and require a substantial fee to access. Open access journals are changing this model by making articles available for free to anyone who wants to read them; however, they do this by passing the cost of publication to the author (many open access journals can cost upwards of $2,000 to publish in).

Once people have access to an article, they may find the article dense, jargonistic, and difficult to understand (after all, journal articles are typically written for other scholars and not a general audience). Santos (2012: 244) writes that "activists do not engage with the existing literature on the sociology of social movements, opting instead for reading history biographies and memoirs." In other words, the people you might most want to reach may never have the benefit of your work.

Aside from writing for a scientific audience, we can think about ways to communicate our findings to groups outside of academia. For example, we might consider writing opinion pieces and editorials, writing for patients and their caregivers, writing a book for a trade press, writing a white paper, writing text for a health application, or putting together arts-based representations such as poetry or ethnodrama. There are many outlets we can use to write for the public.

When writing for a general audience, inspect the language that you use. Generally, you want to write at approximately a fifth-grade level. If your word processing program doesn't have a tool for evaluating the reading level of your writing, you can find one for free on the internet. If you must use jargon, define the terms with clear wording. In addition, consider how long it will take someone to read your work, and keep it as brief as possible. Many people will stop reading if the piece is too long, so make your point quickly.

If you would like to target people who read a different language than what you are writing in, translate your document and ask several native speakers to read it to make sure the translation says what you want it to say.

Voice

Qualitative researchers have two voices to contend with—our own and the voices of our participants. We begin our discussion with authorial voice.

Often, my students tell me that when they read my work, they can hear my voice in their heads. It would be weird to me if they didn't; it would mean that I hadn't written in my voice. Think about the authors that you enjoy reading. Compare them to the articles you skim, you don't finish, or that make you sleepy. If your reader doesn't enjoy reading your work, they won't. How many half-read books do you have on your bookshelf? Why didn't you finish them? What about journal articles that you didn't read all the way through?

Authorial voice is literally the voice that the reader hears while reading. It's ok to let your personality come through. In fact, that is what will keep people reading. Anton Chekhov said, "There are big dogs and little dogs, but little dogs must not fret over the existence of the big ones. Everyone is obligated to howl in the voice that the Lord God has given him" (as quoted in Narayan 2012: 86). Our writing voice is our howl.

For the most part, I write the same way that I talk. I read all of my work out loud. Does it sound like me? Although I will edit for clarity, I don't want to edit out my own voice (nor do I want an editor to do so). Hart (2011: 73) writes, "The ultimate secret to letting your voice sound on the page is simply to relax and be yourself." He continues: "A relaxed writer is a fast writer, and fast writers sound more like themselves . . . Writers who agonize over a rough draft, futzing with every word, will submerge their true selves in nondescript formality." Write fast, edit later.

In qualitative writing, we also have to consider the voices of our participants. They shouldn't sound like us; they should sound like themselves.

As we discussed in Chapter 8, a common refrain among students in the social sciences is that they wish to speak for the voiceless. Let's abolish that phrase from our vocabulary right now. No one is voiceless. It is true, however, that some people have the power to amplify their voice, whereas others do not. This is an important distinction. Stringer (1999: 39) writes that "the voices of the most powerless groups tend to go unheard, their agendas ignored, and their needs unmet." If you hold the power of amplification (which we as academics do), it is important to know when to speak and when to "pass the mic" to others whose voices are silenced.

In the 1990s, during what have been called the "science wars" and the "crisis of representation," social scientists debated this question of being the voice of the voiceless. The crisis of representation involves the question of who has the right to speak for someone else (Gullion 2018). Some researchers argued that interpretation of people's lives by outsiders is a form of violence against them. Linda Smith (2012: 8) writes,

> Research is one of the ways in which the underlying code of imperialism and colonialism is both regulated and realized. It is regulated through the formal rules of individual scholarly disciplines and scientific paradigms, and the institutions that support them (including the state). It is realized in the myriad of representations and ideological constructions of the Other in scholarly and "popular" works, and in the principles which help to select and recontextualize those constructions in such things as the media, official histories and school curricula.

When we conduct research, there are systems of power we must be mindful of. What systems of power are at play here? How does your writing reveal or support those systems of power?

When we do research (whether it is qualitative or quantitative), we interrupt people's lives and ask something of them. Their opinion, their stories, or our wanting to watch them engage in something they are doing. Most of the time, we leave and that's the end of our relationship with them.

In some cases, we don't even have that much contact with people. We might conduct secondary data analysis—that is, using information that someone else collected for some other purpose and writing a paper from it. Thus, we end up with someone who's an expert on substance abuse without ever having talked with an addict, or someone who is an expert on Venezuela without ever having been there.

That seems awfully arrogant, and some researchers argue it is a form of violence and a theft of knowledge. This is where the crisis of representation comes from—self-defined experts speaking *for* a group of people rather than using their social capital to amplify the voices of the group members.

When thinking about research in lieu of the crisis of representation, we must ask what gives someone the right to speak for others. Does having a PhD alone confer someone that right? Often, the people whose voices are silenced are also pathologized. Assumptions are made by people in power, and actions are taken on behalf of the silenced, without ever consulting them.

Standpoint theory (D. Smith 1974) tells us that we all have our own perspectives on reality and truth, which are grounded in the intersections of our identities and experiences. Given this, conceptualization of constructs such as reality and truth can differ from person to person. Issues of power come into play when one person's truth is elevated above someone else's. This is not necessarily a bad thing. One truth could be informed by all sorts of evidence, the other not. Conceptualizations of reality and truth are therefore not equal or equally valid to whatever specific situation is at hand.

When conducting research, we need to consider the various voices involved in any particular conversation, especially those that have been silenced and/or pathologized, because they may hold the answer to our problem. At the same time, we need to be aware that the words we hear are always only a partial representation of a phenomena in question. MacLure (2009: 101) writes,

> Subjects might always have said something more, or something else, or something deeper, or something more true—if they had felt more at ease; if they had been more honest; if the researcher had asked better questions; or had "shared" more of herself; or introjected less of herself; if the interview had been in a less public place; or a more public place; if it had taken place in a group; or had *not* taken place in a group; if the subject and researcher had been the same sex, or age, or ethnicity, and so on. There is no "perfect" interview. Interviewing is relational, a co-creation of knowledge that occurs during a (typically unusual) encounter.

Jackson and Mazzei (2009: 1–2) write that qualitative researchers have a romantic notion of voice. We tend to rely on specific words spoken to use in the course of our research as Truth (with a capital T). We record interviews, transcribe them, analyze them, and (re)present them as fact. Yet, Jackson and Mazzei note, voice is unstable. Mutable. Voice changes based on the situation. It changes based on who we are speaking to. It changes because of all sorts of variables. The story I tell you today is not exactly the same as the one I told yesterday, nor that I will tell about this event in the future. Yet researchers will transubstantiate words generated during research into concrete data.

Jackson and Mazzei (2009) invite us to problematize voice and representation—that we consider when we are the appropriate person to speak and when it is appropriate for us to be silent. So let's talk about how to include participants' voices in our writing.

As I said earlier, their voices should sound like their voices. This means you need to consider if you will (or to what extent you will) edit what they said. I once had an editor try to change a participant's words when he said a colloquialism the editor had never heard before. The editor noted, "Surely there is a better way to say this." Surely there was, but if I changed the quote, I would erase the quirkiness of my participant. Why would I want to do that? That being said, we don't want to embarrass our participants. Hart (2011: 86) reminds us that "speech itself is a status indicator." One way to help you with this is to do member checks when you write about people. Show them what you've written and ask them if you are representing them properly.

I mentioned earlier that ethics should continue beyond the IRB. We need to be ethical in our writing as well. We need to question what and whose reality we are representing in our writing. We need to ask how accurate and how trustworthy our words are. If you presented your writing to the people you researched with, what would they say about what you've written? How would your words make them feel? Are your words empowering or disempowering? Although the answers to these questions may differ project to project, you need to ask them of your work.

Some researchers have moved to autoethnography as the only ethical response to this crisis. Autoethnographers center themselves in their research. Through writing as inquiry (Richardson 2009), and using one's own experiences as data, a researcher explores the intersection of history with their own biography (Mills 1959).

First, Second, or Third Person

For some reason I cannot fathom, schoolchildren are taught to write in third person. My daughter, who was in middle school at the time, asked me to look over a paper she'd written for her English class about gun control. Through the whole thing, she spoke about herself as "the author." I had her change all that to "I" and "me," and then she ended up failing the paper because the teacher insisted on third person (this is one of the many reasons I should stay away from my children's homework. I also got in trouble with several math teachers for teaching them the "easy way" instead of Common Core).

Writing in third person takes away your authority. It's an attempt to take an omniscient overview of the writing. Some people like this; they don't want to take responsibility for their thoughts. I think you should own your thoughts. It's your work, and you should stand by it. "The researcher" didn't find these things, you did.

We rarely write in second person. That's usually reserved for things such as textbooks, when I as the author address you, the reader, directly.

These are general guidelines, however. You may find a particular story needs to be written in second or third person; that's ok. But try writing in first person and see how that works out for you. In addition to owning your own work, writing that is in first person is easier to read. It is more likely to use active voice rather than passive. My mentor used to slam me for writing in passive voice. She would circle every instance of "is," "was," "to be," and other passive verbs and tell me to rewrite the sentence with active verbs instead. "Active voice," Hart (2011: 115) writes, "advances the narrative by showing why and how human beings affect the world around them." As you research through your writing, make sure that you identify who is doing the action and what that action is. Here is an example:

Passive: Coding was done using qualitative data analytic software.
Active: I coded the data using qualitative data analytic software.

And please avoid writing, "This paper does . . . ." Because this paper does nothing. It's a piece of paper. Instead, in this paper, *you* are doing something. You are the actor, not the paper. Becker (1986: 8) notes that passive voice also dilutes your theoretical argument: "If you say, for example, that 'deviants were labeled,' you don't have to say who labeled them. That is a theoretical error, not just bad writing." The persons doing the labeling are important to labeling theory. We can't leave them out. They tell us who has power in the relationship and who doesn't.

Big Words Don't Mean You're Smart

Big words and convoluted prose do not make you sound smarter. This is a common misunderstanding among academics, who think they must pontificate to impress their peers.

It's ok to use jargon with the right audience. When I write for my qualitative peers, I use words such as triangulation and epistemology because I know they know what those words mean. They understand the context. I can throw the same words around in a different setting and sound like a pompous jerk.

Jargon often gets in the way of the readability of your work. And after all the work you put into it, don't you want people to read it? C. Wright Mills (1959: 218–219, as quoted in Becker 1986: 31) writes that the

> lack of ready intelligibility [in scholarly writing], I believe, usually has little or nothing to do with the complexity of the subject matter, and nothing at all to do with the profundity of thought. It has to do almost entirely with certain confusions of the academic writer about his [sic] own status. . . . To overcome the academic *prose* you have to overcome the academic *post*.

Of course we want people to think we are smart, we are academics after all. But we don't want to fill our writing with "polysyllabic bullshit" (Becker 1986: 10) either.

Saldaña (2011: 141) advocates for elegance in writing:

> Elegance means *simplicity*. Writing that is elegant relies on trusting the power of the research tale itself; told in a clear and straightforward manner. You needn't try to impress anyone with convoluted prose. It is most often the *ideas* that will make a lasting impact and impression on your reader.

If you can put forth your ideas in a way that is both interesting and understandable to your reader, they are more likely to keep reading. And ultimately, that's what we want.

Editing

I have provided you a lot of advice about writing, but we need to also talk about how to edit. I find that many writers focus on the writing of their work, without expending as much time editing. Ideally, you should spend half your time writing and half your time editing.

No writer, not even the most famous writers you can think of, gets everything correct on their first pass. In fact, a lot of what they initially write might be garbage and get cut later. The good news about this is that you don't have to stress over every word you put on the page. No one ever has to see your first draft, and you can edit later.

If you have time, it is helpful to put your document away for a few weeks after you've written it. That will help you see it fresh. Work on something else and take your mind off it. This also helps you read what is actually on the page as opposed to what you *meant* to say.

Once you decide it is time to edit, you must attend to three levels of editing: the overall structure of the piece, the individual sentences, and the citations.

We begin with the overall structure of the piece. To do this, I usually create a detailed outline of whatever it is I am working on. I then take a look at it to see if it makes logical sense. Remember when we talked about story arcs earlier? Consider the arc of whatever piece you are writing. You may find that you need to move things around some. That's ok; do what you need to do for the order of things to make sense. You might also find that you've left something important out, some between step or connection, or some topic that will help round out the narrative. Add that in.

Think about the main point you are trying to make with this piece. Did you make it? Or does it get lost in your prose? "Every book—at least every one worth reading—is about *something*." King (2000: 201) writes,

> Your job during or just after the first draft is to decide what something or somethings yours is about. Your job in the second draft—or one of them, anyway—is to make that something even more clear. This may necessitate some big changes and revisions. The benefits to you and your reader will be clearer focus and a more unified story.

After the structure is sound, it is time for you to examine each sentence. This can get tedious, I know, but it is worth it. You're looking for sentences that don't make sense, that have grammatical errors, that run on too long, or that aren't long enough. Sentences that are in passive voice. Sentences in which it is not clear who or what is doing the action. Look for words that you should have defined for your reader. And fix all your typos.

To be a good writer, you must understand writing. Grammar, sentence structure, vocabulary—all of the words on the page must have a reason for existing there. Too many academics may be good researchers but are terrible writers. "Sentences have skeletons," Le Guin and Naimon (2018: 21) note, and you must understand how those skeletons hang together.

I have found that reading the piece out loud can help you catch some of those mistakes. If you can't get through a sentence without taking a breath, maybe you need a comma. Or maybe the sentence is too long. If you stumble over the words, change them. If you find yourself getting bored, figure out what is wrong and fix that. I've also found that I catch other problems when I print out my document and look at it on paper as opposed to a screen. For some reason, when I see mistakes on the screen, my brain will sometimes read them as I meant to write them and not as they are actually written.

Another suggestion is to read your paper backwards. Not literally. But start with the last paragraph and read it in isolation. Then read the second to last paragraph. And so on. This takes your sentences out of context so you can examine them as they stand on their own.

Next, check to see that all of your in-text citations have references and that all references have in-text citations. Use the "find" function in your word processing program to make this go faster. Double-check that quotes have page numbers and that all your references are formatted correctly. Check for drifts in authors' last names. I once wrote a paper citing a person named Johnston a lot and about halfway through the paper changed the person's name to Johnson. Fortunately, one of the reviewers caught it, because I hadn't.

Once you think the work is finished, show it to someone you trust to give you helpful, honest feedback. Students should ask their mentors for help. Tenured faculty will usually help junior faculty with this. They may catch something that you missed.

I have two caveats to this suggestion. The first is that when you show your piece to others, don't take their feedback personally. Their critique is not a critique of you as a person. Instead, they are giving you suggestions on how to improve your writing. Use what you find helpful.

Second, forget perfectionism. More than once I have had to tell a student their dissertation was good enough and force them to turn it in. "Perfection is the voice of the oppressor," Lamott (1995: 28) writes, "the enemy of the people. It will keep you cramped and insane your whole life." If you are ever going to be a published writer, you need to send your work out for publication. Even if you are not one hundred percent sure it's ready.

Writing is an embodied practice. One must sit down, pen in hand, or typing on keys, or dictating orally. There is a doing that must occur that requires both body and discourse. Many people want to have written, to see their name in print. But to have written, one must write first. One must do the work.

References

Becker, Howard S. 1986. *Writing for Social Scientists: How to Start and Finish Your Thesis, Book, or Article.* Chicago: University of Chicago Press.

Denzin, Norman K. 2010. *The Qualitative Manifesto: A Call to Arms.* Walnut Creek, CA: Left Coast Press.

Faulkner, Sandra L. 2020. *Poetic Inquiry: Craft, Method and Practice*, 2nd ed. London: Routledge.

Grudniewicz, Agnes, David Moher, Kelly D. Cobey, Gregory L. Bryson, Samantha Cukier, Kristiann Allen, Clear Ardern, et al. 2019. "Predatory Journals: No Definition, No Defense." *Nature* 576: 210–212.

Gullion, Jessica Smartt. 2018. *Diffractive Ethnography: Social Sciences in the Ontological Turn.* London: Routledge.

Hart, Jack. 2011. *Storycraft: The Complete Guide to Writing Narrative Nonfiction.* Chicago: University of Chicago Press.

Jackson, Alecia Y., and Lisa A. Mazzei. 2009. *Voice in Qualitative Inquiry: Challenging Conventional, Interpretive, and Critical Conceptions in Qualitative Research.* New York: Routledge.

King, Stephen. 2000. *On Writing: A Memoir of the Craft.* New York: Pocket Books.

Lamott, Anne. 1995. *Bird by Bird: Some Instructions on Writing and Life.* New York: Anchor.

Leavy, Patricia. 2020. *Method Meets Art: Arts-Based Research Practice*, 3rd ed. New York: Guilford.

Le Guin, Ursula K., and David Naimon. 2018. *Conversations on Writing.* Portland, OR: Tin House Books.

MacLure, Maggie. 2009. "Broken Voices, Dirty Words." In *Voice in Qualitative Inquiry: Challenging Conventional, Interpretive, and Critical Conceptions in Qualitative Research*, edited by Alecia Y. Jackson and Lisa A. Mazzei, 97–113. New York: Routledge.

Mills, C. Wright. 1959. *The Sociological Imagination.* New York: Oxford University Press.

Narayan, Kirin. 2012. *Alive in the Writing: Crafting Ethnography in the Company of Chekhov.* Chicago: University of Chicago Press.

Richardson, Laurel. 2009. "Writing Theory in(to) Last Writes." In *Ethnographies Revisited: Constructing Theory in the Field*, edited by Antony J. Puddephatt, William Shaffir, and Steven W. Kleinknocht, 307–317. London: Routledge.

Saldaña, Johnny. 2011. *Fundamentals of Qualitative Research*. New York: Oxford University Press.
Santos, Ana Cristina. 2012. "Disclosed and Willing: Towards a Queer Public Sociology." *Social Movement Studies* 11, no. 2: 241–254.
Smith, Dorothy E. 1974. "Women's Perspective as a Radical Critique of Sociology." *Sociological Inquiry* 44, no. 1: 7–13.
Smith, Linda Tuhiwai. 2012. *Decolonizing Methodologies: Research and Indigenous Peoples*, 2nd ed. London: Zed Books.
Stringer, Ernest T. 1999. *Action Research*, 2nd ed. Thousand Oaks, CA: SAGE.

Further Reading

Behar, Ruth. 1997. *The Vulnerable Observer: Anthropology That Breaks Your Heart*. Boston: Beacon.
Cameron, Julia. 1992. *The Artist's Way*. New York: Tarcher.
Goldberg, Natalie. 2006. *Writing Down the Bones: Freeing the Writer Within*. Boulder, CO: Shambhala.

Discussion Questions

1. Why is voice important?
2. How do you get something published in an academic journal?

Active Learning

1. Revise a paper that you have written for voice. For example, if the paper is in third person, write it in first person. Notice the differences in the two pieces.
2. Review a classmate's work as if you were a peer reviewer for a journal. Would you publish it? Write an honest critical review of their work, and give them advice on how to improve it.

Mindfulness Exercises

1. How did you learn how to write?
2. Under what conditions do you write best (e.g., in a coffee shop, after you've cleaned the kitchen)?

Glossary

analysis	The examination of a complex subject.
bias	Influencing the outcome of research to reflect what you want it to, rather than what you found.
coding	The process of reducing data into categories and themes.
content analysis	A technique for studying documents or other artifacts produced by humans.
data	The empirical materials of research.
deductive	Reasoning that derives testable hypotheses from theory.
empirical materials	The flotsam and jetsam on which research is based.
epidemiology	The study of disease in a population.
epistemology	The study of how we know things; how things become "true."
ethnography	Observation and participation in a group of people to understand their culture.
experiment	A scientific procedure for testing theory; normally an experimental group is compared with a control group (non-experimental group) to determine if there is any difference between the two groups.
field notes	Written accounts of observations that occurred during data collection.
focus groups	Interviews with a group of people that seek to form group synergy.
inductive	Reasoning based on the collection of data.
inquiry	The process of seeking information about a subject of interest.
memos	Notes a researcher keeps about the theoretical aspects of their research and findings.
method	The technique a researcher uses to collect data.
methodology	The study of research methods.
neoliberal	Valuing free market capitalism and deregulation; restructuring universities to run like businesses, with a focus on return on investment.
objectivity	The idea that a researcher holds no preconceived notions about the research or possible outcomes of the study.
ontology	The study of reality and of what is real.
othered/othering	The idea that a group of people are not like the group you belong to; the belief that your group is superior.
positivism	A philosophical system that exerts that an external reality exists which is measurable and knowable.
post-positivism	A critique of positivism's notion that an external reality exists.

post-qualitative	Qualitative inquiry that explores ontology rather than focusing on epistemology.
qualitative methods	Research methods that use words, sounds, images, and other non-numerical artifacts as data.
quantitative methods	Research methods that use numbers as data.
questionnaire	A list of questions used in interviewing.
reflexivity	The practice of examining how one's standpoint influences one's research.
reliability	Getting the same results every time an instrument is used.
research methods	The techniques used to gather and analyze data for research purposes.
research question	The main problem of a research project; the overriding reason for doing the research.
rigor/rigorous	The trustworthiness of the study.
saturation	The point at which adding additional information does not have an impact on the research findings.
social science	The study of society and individuals within a society.
standpoint	The totality of a person's identities and experiences.
survey	A list of questions, the majority of which have predefined answers the research participant selects from.
systematic	Using a defined method or technique.
theory	An explanation about some aspect of the social or natural world.
triangulation	The use of multiple research methods to answer a research question.
unit of analysis	The "thing" under investigation—for example, groups of individuals or phenomena.
validity	The degree to which your study represents the real world.

References

American Association of University Professors. 2000. "Institutional Review Boards and Social Science Research." Accessed November 20, 2019. https://www.aaup.org/report/institutional-review-boards-and-social-science-research.

Anderson, Patrick. 2017. *Autobiography of a Disease*. New York: Routledge.

Arndt, Sonja. 2017. "(Un)becoming Data Through Philosophical Thought Processes of Pasts, Presents and Futures." In *Disrupting Data in Qualitative Inquiry: Entanglements with the Post-Critical and Post-Anthropocentric*, edited by Mirka Koro-Ljungberg, Teija Löytönen, and Marek Tesar, 93–104. New York: Lang.

Atkinson, Paul, Amanda Coffey, Sara Delamont, John Lofland, and Lyn Lofland. 2001. *Handbook of Ethnography*. Los Angeles: SAGE.

Baker, Max B. 2014. "Texas Town Bans Fracking in the Heart of Texas Oil Country." *Fort Worth Star-Telegram*. https://www.star-telegram.com/news/politics-government/article3906359.html.

Baker, Shamim M., Otis W. Brawley, and Leonard S. Marks. 2005. "Effects of Untreated Syphilis in the Negro Male, 1932 to 1972: A Closure Comes to the Tuskegee Study, 2004." *Urology* 65, no. 6: 1259–1262.

Barad, Karen. 2007. *Meeting the Universe Halfway: Quantum Physics and the Entanglement of Matter and Meaning*. Durham, NC: Duke University Press.

Barad, Karen. 2014. "Diffracting Diffraction: Cutting Together-Apart." *Parallax* 20, no. 3: 168–187.

Beck, Ulrich, and Elizabeth Beck-Gernsheim. 2002. *Individualization: Institutional Individualism and Its Social and Political Consequences*. Thousand Oaks, CA: SAGE.

Becker, Howard S. 1986. *Writing for Social Scientists: How to Start and Finish Your Thesis, Book, or Article*. Chicago: University of Chicago Press.

Bhattacharya, Kakali. 2007. "Consenting to the Consent Form: What Are the Fixed and Fluid Understandings Between the Researcher and the Researched?" *Qualitative Inquiry* 13, no. 8: 1095–1115.

Bhattacharya, Kakali, and Jeong-Hee Kim. 2018. "Reworking Prejudice in Qualitative Inquiry with Gadamer and De/Colonizing Onto-Epistemologies." *Qualitative Inquiry* 24, no. 3: 1–10.

Bourdieu, Pierre. 1983. "Forms of Capital." In *Handbook of Theory and Research for the Sociology of Education*, edited by John G. Richardson, 241–258. New York: Greenwood.

Boyton, Marcella H., David B. Portnoy, and Blair T. Johnson. 2013. "Exploring the Ethics and Psychological Impact of Deception in Psychological Research." *IRB* 35, no. 2: 7–13.

Burawoy, Michael. 1998. "The Extended Case Method." *Sociological Theory* 16, no. 1: 4–33.

Butler-Kisber, Lynn. 2010. *Qualitative Inquiry: Thematic, Narrative and Arts-Informed Perspectives*. Los Angeles: SAGE.

Charmaz, Kathy. 2010. "Studying the Experience of Chronic Illness Through Grounded Theory." In *New Directions in the Sociology of Chronic and Disabling Conditions: Assaults on the Lifeworld*, edited by Graham Scambler and Sasha Scambler, 8–36. London: Palgrave.

Charmaz, Kathy. 2014. *Constructing Grounded Theory*, 2nd ed. Los Angeles: SAGE.

Charmaz, Kathy, Robert Thornberg, and Elaine Keane. 2018. "Evolving Grounded Theory and Social Justice Inquiry." In *The SAGE Handbook of Qualitative Research*, 5th ed., edited by Norman K. Denzin and Yvonna S. Lincoln, 411–443. Thousand Oaks, CA: SAGE.

Clarke, Adele E. 2005. *Situational Analysis: Grounded Theory After the Postmodern Turn*. Los Angeles: SAGE.

Davis, Charlotte Aull. 2008. *Reflexive Ethnography: A Guide to Researching Selves and Others*, 2nd ed. New York: Routledge.

Deegan, Mary Jo. 2001. "The Chicago School of Ethnography." In *Handbook of Ethnography*, edited by Paul Atkinson, Amanda Coffey, Sara Delamont, John Lofland, and Lyn Lofland, 11–25. London: SAGE.

Denzin, Norman K. 2010. *The Qualitative Manifesto: A Call to Arms*. Walnut Creek, CA: Left Coast Press.

Denzin, Norman K. 2017. "Data: The Wonder of It All." In *Disrupting Data in Qualitative Inquiry: Entanglements with the Post-Critical and Post-Anthropocentric*, edited by Mirka Koro-Ljungberg, Teija Löytönen, and Marek Tesar, 81–91. New York: Lang.

Denzin, Norman K., and Yvonna S. Lincoln. 2018. "Introduction: The Discipline and Practice of Qualitative Research." In *The SAGE Handbook of Qualitative Research*, 5th ed., edited by Norman K. Denzin and Yvonna S. Lincoln, 1–26. Los Angeles: SAGE.

DuBois, W. E. B. 1899. *The Philadelphia Negro: A Social Study*. Philadelphia: University of Pennsylvania Press.

Duhn, Iris. 2017. "Performing Data." In *Disrupting Data in Qualitative Inquiry: Entanglements with the Post-Critical and Post-Anthropocentric*, edited by Mirka Koro-Ljungberg, Teija Löytönen, and Marek Tesar, 11–21. New York: Lang.

Durkheim, Emile. 1895/1982. *The Rules of Sociological Method*, translated by W. D. Halls. New York: Free Press.

Ellingson, Laura L. 2017. *Embodiment in Qualitative Research*. New York: Routledge.

Ellis, Carolyn. 2007. "Telling Secrets, Revealing Lives: Relational Ethics in Research with Intimate Others." *Qualitative Inquiry* 13, no. 1: 3–29.

Ellis, Erin. 2020. "Giving Birth in the Ivory Tower: A Closer Look at the Unique Needs of Pregnant and Parenting Graduate Student Mothers." Doctoral dissertation.

Erdley, Deb. 2011. "Ex-Pitt Professor Given Sanctions for Plagiarism." TribLIVE. Accessed September 11, 2019. https://archive.triblive.com/news/ex-pitt-professor-given-sanctions-for-plagiarism.

Erickson, Frederick. 2018. "A History of Qualitative Inquiry in Social Science and Educational Research." In The SAGE Handbook of Qualitative Research, 5th ed., edited by Norman K. Denzin and Yvonna S. Lincoln, 36–65. Los Angeles: SAGE.

Eveleth, Rose. 2014. "Academic Write Papers Arguing Over How Many People Read (and Cite) Their Papers." *Smithsonian Magazine*. Accessed January 31, 2020. https://www.smithsonianmag.com/smart-news/half-academic-studies-are-never-read-more-three-people-180950222.

Faulkner, Sandra L. 2020. *Poetic Inquiry: Craft, Method and Practice*, 2nd ed. London: Routledge.

Fox, Nick J., and Pam Alldred. 2017. *Sociology and the New Materialism: Theory, Research, Action*. Los Angeles: SAGE.

Gane, Nicholas. 2011. "Measure, Value, and the Current Crisis in Sociology." *Sociological Review* 59, no. 2: 151–173.

Gaudry, Adam J. 2011. "Insurgent Research." *Wicazo Sa Review* 26, no. 1: 113–136.

Gaukroger, Stephen. 2012. *Objectivity: A Very Short Introduction*. New York: Oxford University Press.

Geertz, Clifford. 1973. "Thick Description: Toward an Interpretive Theory of Culture." In *The Interpretation of Cultures: Selected Essays*, edited by Clifford Geertz, 3–30. New York: Basic Books.

Glaser, Barney G., and Anselm L. Strauss. 1967. *The Discovery of Grounded Theory: Strategies for Qualitative Research*. Chicago: Aldine.

Golden-Biddle, Karen, and Karen Locke. 2007. *Composing Qualitative Research*, 2nd ed. Thousand Oaks, CA: SAGE.

Goodman, Howard. 1998. "Studying Prison Experiment Research: For 20 Years, a Dermatologist Used the Inmates of a Philadelphia Prison as the Willing Subjects of Tests on Shampoo, Foot Powder, Deodorant, and Later, Mind-Altering Drugs and Dioxin." *The Baltimore Sun*. Accessed September 11, 2020. https://www.baltimoresun.com/news/bs-xpm-1998-07-21-1998202099-story.html.

Grudniewicz, Agnes, David Moher, Kelly D. Cobey, Gregory L. Bryson, Samantha Cukier, Kristiann Allen, Clear Ardern, et al. 2019. "Predatory Journals: No Definition, No Defense." *Nature* 576: 210–212.

Gullion, Jessica Smartt. 2004. "School Nurses as Volunteers in a Bioterrorism Event." *Biosecurity and Bioterrorism* 2, no. 2: 112–117.

Gullion, Jessica Smartt. 2008. "Scholar, Negated." In *Mama, PhD: Women Write About Motherhood and Academic Life*, edited by Elrena Evans and Caroline Grant, 16–19. New Brunswick, NJ: Rutgers University Press.

Gullion, Jessica Smartt. 2013. "Toxic Neighborhood." *Qualitative Inquiry* 19, no. 7: 491–492.

Gullion, Jessica Smartt. 2014. "This Toxic Material: A Poetic (Re)Presentation of Cancer/Environmental Assemblages." *International Review of Qualitative Research* 7, no. 4: 401–420.

Gullion, Jessica Smartt. 2015. *Fracking the Neighborhood: Reluctant Activists and Natural Gas Drilling*. Cambridge, MA: MIT Press.

Gullion, Jessica Smartt. 2016. *Writing Ethnography*. Rotterdam, the Netherlands: Sense Publishers.

Gullion, Jessica Smartt. 2018. *Diffractive Ethnography: Social Sciences in the Ontological Turn*. London: Routledge.

Gullion, Jessica Smartt. 2022. *Writing Ethnography*, 2nd ed. Leiden, the Netherlands: Brill.

Gullion, Jessica Smartt, and Abigail Tilton. 2020. *Researching with: A Decolonizing Approach to Community-Based Action Research*. Rotterdam, the Netherlands: Brill/Sense.

Halse, Christine, and Anne Honey. 2007. "Rethinking Ethics Review as Institutional Discourse." *Qualitative Inquiry* 13, no. 3: 336–352.

Halseth, Greg, Sean Markey, Laura Ryser, and Don Manson. 2016. *Doing Community-Based Research: Perspectives from the Field*. Montreal, Quebec, Canada: McGill-Queen's University Press.

Harper, Krista, and Aline Gubrium. 2017. "Visual and Multimodal Approaches in Anthropological Participatory Action Research." *General Anthropology* 24, no. 2: 1–8.

Hart, Jack. 2011. *Storycraft: The Complete Guide to Writing Narrative Nonfiction*. Chicago: University of Chicago Press.

Heinkel-Wolfe, Peggy. 2014, November 5. "Fracking Banned." *Denton Record-Chronicle*.

Humble, Áine M., and M. Elise Radina. 2019. *How Qualitative Data Analysis Happens: Moving Beyond "Themes Emerged."* London: Routledge.

Humphreys, Laud. 1975. *Tearoom Trade: Impersonal Sex in Public Places*. New York: Routledge.

Jackson, Alecia Y., and Lisa A. Mazzei. 2009. *Voice in Qualitative Inquiry: Challenging Conventional, Interpretive, and Critical Conceptions in Qualitative Research*. New York: Routledge.

Jackson, Alecia Y., and Lisa A. Mazzei. 2012. *Thinking with Theory in Qualitative Research: Viewing Data Across Multiple Perspectives*. New York: Routledge.

Jordan, Dian. 2020. *Art in the Community: The Harold Stevenson Collection*. Idabell, OK: The Museum of the Red River.

King, Charles. 2019. *Gods of the Upper Air: How a Circle of Renegade Anthropologists Reinvented Race, Sex, and Gender in the Twentieth Century*. New York: Doubleday.

King, Stephen. 2000. *On Writing: A Memoir of the Craft*. New York: Pocket Books.

Kirby, Vicki. 2011. *Quantum Anthropologies: Life at Large*. Durham, NC: Duke University Press.

Konnikova, Maria. 2015. "The Real Lesson of the Stanford Prison Experiment." *The New Yorker*. Accessed June 6, 2020. https://www.newyorker.com/science/maria-konnikova/the-real-lesson-of-the-stanford-prison-experiment.

Koro-Ljungberg, Mirka, Teija Löytönen, and Marek Tesar. 2017. "Introduction: Multiplicities of Data Encounters." In *Disrupting Data in Qualitative Inquiry: Entanglements with the Post-Critical and Post-Anthropocentric*, edited by Mirka Koro-Ljungberg, Teija Löytönen, and Marek Tesar, 1–9. New York: Lang.

Kozinets, Robert V. 2020. *Netnography: The Essential Guide to Qualitative Social Media Research*, 3rd ed. Los Angeles: SAGE.

Kuntz, Aaron M. 2019. *Qualitative Inquiry, Cartography, and the Promise of Material Change*. London: Routledge.

Lamott, Anne. 1995. *Bird by Bird: Some Instructions on Writing and Life*. New York: Anchor.

Landsberger, Henry A. 1957. *Hawthorne Revisited: A Plea for an Open City*. Ithaca, NY: Cornell University Press.

Lapadat, Judith C. 2018. "Collaborative Autoethnography: An Ethical Approach to Inquiry That Makes a Difference." In *Qualitative Inquiry in the Public Sphere*, edited by Norman K. Denzin and Michael D. Giardina, 156–170. New York: Routledge.

Lather, Patti. 2009. *Engaging Science Policy: From the Side of the Messy*. New York: Lang.

Latour, Bruno. 2005. *Reassembling the Social: An Introduction to Actor-Network-Theory*. Oxford, UK: Oxford University Press.

Latz, Amanda O. 2017. *Photovoice Research in Education and Beyond: A Practical Guide from Theory to Exhibition*. New York: Routledge.

Leavy, Patricia. 2020. *Method Meets Art: Arts-Based Research Practice*, 3rd ed. New York: Guilford.

Le Guin, Ursula K., and David Naimon. 2018. *Conversations on Writing*. Portland, OR: Tin House Books.

MacDonald, Sharon. 2001. "British Social Anthropology." In *Handbook of Ethnography*, edited by Paul Atkinson, Amanda Coffey, Sara Delamont, John Lofland, and Lyn Lofland, 60–79. Los Angeles: SAGE.

MacLure, Maggie. 2009. "Broken Voices, Dirty Words." In *Voice in Qualitative Inquiry: Challenging Conventional, Interpretive, and Critical Conceptions in Qualitative Research*, edited by Alecia Y. Jackson and Lisa A. Mazzei, 97–113. New York: Routledge.

Madden, Raymond. 2010. *Being Ethnographic: A Guide to the Theory and Practice of Ethnography*. Los Angeles: SAGE.

Malinowski, Bronislaw. 1922/2016. *Argonauts of the Western Pacific: An Account of Native Enterprise and Adventure in the Archipelagos of Melanesia New Guinea*. London: Oxford University Press.

Malinsky, Lynn, Ruth DuBois, and Diane Jacquest. 2010. "Building Scholarship Capacity and Transforming the Nurse Educator's Practice Through Institutional Ethnography." *International Journal of Nursing Education Scholarship* 7, no. 1: 1–12.

Mardiros, Marilyn. 2001. "Reconnecting Communities Through Community-Based Action Research." *International Journal of Mental Health* 30, no. 2: 58–78.

Marker, Michael. 2009. "Indigenous Voice, Community, and Epistemic Violence: The Ethnographer's 'Interests' and What 'Interests' the Ethnographer." In *Voice in Qualitative Inquiry: Challenging Conventional, Interpretive, and Critical Conceptions in Qualitative Research*, edited by Alecia Y. Jackson and Lisa A. Mazzei, 27–43. New York: Routledge.

Maron, Dina Fine. 2014. "Should Prisoners Be Used in Medical Experiments?" *Scientific American*. Accessed September 11, 2020. https://www.scientificamerican.com/article/should-prisoners-be-used-in-medical-experiments.

Maynes, Mary Jo, Jennifer L. Piece, and Barbara Laslett. 2008. *Telling Stories: The Use of Personal Narratives in the Social Sciences and History*. Ithaca, NY: Cornell University Press.

McCambridge, Jim, John Witton, and Diana R. Elbourne. 2014. "Systematic Review of the Hawthorne Effect: New Concepts Are Needed to Study Research Participation Effects." *Journal of Clinical Epidemiology* 67, no. 3: 267–277.

Merton, Robert K. 1949. *Social Theory and Social Structure*. New York: Simon & Schuster.

Mills, C. Wright. 1959. *The Sociological Imagination*. New York: Oxford University Press.

Mol, Annemarie. 2003. *The Body Multiple: Ontology in Medical Practice*. Durham, NC: Duke University Press.

Moreira, Telma, Daphne C. Hernandez, Claudia W. Scott, Rosenda Murillo, Elizabeth M. Vaughan, and Craig A. Johnston. 2018. "*Susto, Coraje, y Fatalismo*: Cultural-Bound Beliefs and the Treatment of Diabetes Among Socioeconomically Disadvantaged Hispanics." *American Journal of Lifestyle Medicine* 12, no. 1: 30–33.

Morris, Alan. 2015. *A Practical Introduction to In-Depth Interviewing*. Los Angeles: SAGE.

Moxley, David P., and Olivia G. M. Washington. 2013. "Helping Older African American Homeless Women Get and Stay out of Homelessness: Reflections on Lessons Learned from Long-Haul Developmental Action Research." *Journal of Progressive Human Services* 24, no. 2: 140–164.

Mulrennan, Monica E., Rodney Mark, and Colin H. Short. 2012. "Revamping Community-Based Conservation Through Participatory Research." *The Canadian Geographer* 56, no. 2: 243–259.

Narayan, Kirin. 2012. *Alive in the Writing: Crafting Ethnography in the Company of Chekhov*. Chicago: University of Chicago Press.

National Archives and Records Administration. 2018. "Common Rule." Accessed September 6, 2020. https://www.ecfr.gov/cgi-bin/retrieveECFR?gp=&SID=83cd09e1c0f5c6937cd9d7513160fc3f&pitd=20180719&n=pt45.1.46&r=PART&ty=HTM.

Olson, Karin. 2011. *Essentials of Qualitative Interviewing*. Walnut Creek, CA: Left Coast Press.

Pandey, Geeta. 2018. "American Killed in India by Endangered Andamans Tribe." BBC News. Accessed November 2018. https://www.bbc.com/news/world-asia-india-46286215.

Pascale, Celine-Marie. 2011. *Cartographies of Knowledge: Exploring Qualitative Epistemologies*. London: SAGE.

Peat, F. David. 2002. *Blackfoot Physics*. Boston: Red Wheel/Weiser.

Phillip, Abby. 2015. "Researcher Who Spiked Rabbit Blood to Fake HIV Vaccine Results Slapped with Rare Prison Sentence." *The Washington Post*. Accessed September 11, 2019. https://www.washingtonpost.com/news/to-your-health/wp/2015/07/01/researcher-who-spiked-rabbit-blood-to-fake-hiv-vaccine-results-slapped-with-rare-prison-sentence.

Phillips, Brenda. 2015. *Mennonite Disaster Service: Building a Therapeutic Community After the Gulf Coast Storms*. New York: Lexington Books.

Pine, Adrienne. 2013. "Revolution as a Care Plan: Ethnography, Nursing, and Somatic Solidarity in Honduras." *Social Science and Medicine* 99: 143–152.

Program for the International Assessment of Adult Competencies. 2013. "Literacy, Numeracy, and Problem Solving in Technology-Rich Environments Among U.S. Adults: Results from the Program for the International Assessment of Adult Competencies 2012." Accessed September 12, 2020. https://nces.ed.gov/pubsearch/pubsinfo.asp?pubid=2014008.

Puddephatt, Antony J., William Shaffir, and Steven W. Kleinknecht. 2009. *Ethnographies Revisited: Constructing Theory in the Field*. London: Routledge.

Reardon, Sara. 2015. "U.S. Vaccine Researcher Sentenced to Prison for Fraud." *Nature* 523: 138–139. https://www.nature.com/news/us-vaccine-researcher-sentenced-to-prison-for-fraud-1.17660?WT.mc_id=TWT_NatureNews.

Reid, Sandra D., Rhoda Reddock, and Tisha Nickenig. 2014. "Breaking the Silence of Child Sexual Abuse in the Caribbean: A Community-Based Action Research Intervention Model." *Journal of Child Sexual Abuse* 23: 256–277.

Renold, Emma, and David Mellor. 2013. "Deleuze and Guattari in the Nursery: Towards a Multi-Sensory Mapping of Young Gendered and Sexual Becomings." In *Deleuze and Research Methodologies*, edited by Rebecca Coleman and Jessica Ringrose, 23–40. Edinburgh, UK: Edinburgh University Press.

Richardson, Laurel. 2009. "Writing Theory in(to) Last Writes." In *Ethnographies Revisited: Constructing Theory in the Field*, edited by Antony J. Puddephatt, William Shaffir, and Steven W. Kleinknocht, 307–317. London: Routledge.

Riordan, Diane A., and Michael P. Riordan. 2009. "IRB Creep: Federal Regulations Protecting Human Research Subjects and Increasing Instructors' Responsibilities." *Issues in Accounting Education* 24, no. 1: 31–43.

Rix, Elizabeth F., Shawn Wilson, Norm Sheehan, and Nicole Tujague. 2018. "Indigenist and Decolonizing Research Methodology." In *Handbook of Research Methods in Health Social Sciences*, edited by Pranee Liamputtong, 1–15. Singapore: Springer.

Rosenblatt, Paul C., and Elizabeth Wieling. 2019. "Thematic and Phenomenological Analysis in Research on Intimate Relationships." In *How Qualitative Data Analysis Happens: Moving Beyond "Themes Emerged,"* edited by Áine H. Humble and M. Elise Radina, 50–63. London: Routledge.

Rowe, Aimee Carrillo, and Eve Tuck. 2016. "Settler Colonialism and Cultural Studies: Ongoing Settlement, Cultural Production, and Resistance." *Cultural Studies ↔ Critical Methodologies* 17, no. 1: 1–11.

Saldaña, Johnny. 2011. *Fundamentals of Qualitative Research*. New York: Oxford University Press.

Saldaña, Johnny. 2016. *The Coding Manual for Qualitative Researchers*, 3rd ed. Los Angeles: SAGE.

Santos, Ana Cristina. 2012. "Disclosed and Willing: Towards a Queer Public Sociology." *Social Movement Studies* 11, no. 2: 241–254.

Savin-Biden, Maggi, and Claire Howell Major. 2013. *Qualitative Research: The Essential Guide to Theory and Practice*. New York: Routledge.

Scheurich, James Joseph. 2018. "Research 4 Revolutionaries by #Jimscheurish." In *Qualitative Inquiry in the Public Sphere*, edited by Norman K. Denzin and Michael D. Giardina, 125–142. New York: Routledge.

Service, Robert F. 2002. "Bell Labs Fires Star Physicist Found Guilty of Forging Data." *Science* 298, no. 5591: 30–31.

Slater, John, and George Ritzer. (2001). "Interview with Urich Beck." *Journal of Consumer Culture*, 1, no. 2: 261–277.

Smith, Dorothy E. 1974. "Women's Perspective as a Radical Critique of Sociology." *Sociological Inquiry* 44, no. 1: 7–13.

Smith, Linda Tuhiwai. 2005. "On Tricky Ground: Researching the Native in the Age of Uncertainty." In *The SAGE Handbook of Qualitative Research*, 4th ed., edited by Norman K. Denzin and Yvonna S. Lincoln, 85–107. Thousand Oaks, CA: SAGE.

Smith, Linda Tuhiwai. 2012. *Decolonizing Methodologies: Research and Indigenous Peoples*, 2nd ed. New York: Zed Books.

St. Pierre, Elizabeth Adams. 2013. "The Appearance of Data." *Cultural Studies ↔ Critical Methodologies* 13, no. 4: 223–227.

Strega, Susan, and Leslie Brown. 2015. *Research as Resistance: Revisiting Critical, Indigenous, and Anti-Oppressive Approaches*, 2nd ed. Toronto: Canadian Scholars' Press.

Stringer, Ernest T. 1999. *Action Research*, 2nd ed. Thousand Oaks, CA: SAGE.

United States Holocaust Memorial Museum. 2006. "Nazi Medical Experiments." Accessed September 6, 2020. https://encyclopedia.ushmm.org/content/en/article/nazi-medical-experiments.

Van Maanen, John. 2011. *Tales of the Field: On Writing Ethnography*, 2nd ed. Chicago: University of Chicago Press.

Vogel, Gretchen. 2011. "Jan Hendrik Schön Loses His Ph.D." *Science*. Accessed September 11, 2019. https://www.sciencemag.org/news/2011/09/jan-hendrik-sch-n-loses-his-phd.

Weaver-Hightower, Marcus B. 2019. "Analyzing Self and Other in Autoethnography." In *How Qualitative Data Analysis Happens: Moving Beyond "Themes Emerged,"* edited by Áine H. Humble and M. Elise Radina, 3–17. London: Routledge.

Weber, Max. 1905/2009. *The Protestant Ethic and the Spirit of Capitalism*, translated by Stephen Kalberg. London: Oxford University Press.

Williamson, Susan, Timothy Twelvetree, Jacqueline Thompson, and Kinta Beaver, 2012. "An Ethnographic Study Exploring the Role of Ward-Based Advanced Nurse Practitioners in an Acute Medical Setting." *Journal of Advanced Nurse Practitioners* 68, no. 7: 1579–1588.

Wolcott, Harry F. 2002. *Sneaky Kid and Its Aftermath: Ethics and Intimacy in Fieldwork*. Walnut Creek, CA: AltaMira.

Zimbardo, Philip G. 1973. "On the Ethics of Intervention in Human Psychological Research: With Special Reference to the Stanford Prison Experiment." *Cognition* 2, no. 2: 243–256.

Index